BIG FAT LIES

The Truth about Obesity, Disease and Health

By: Joey Lott

www.joeylotthealth.com

Publishing services provided by 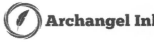 Archangel Ink

ISBN: 1518666485
ISBN-13: 978-1518666483

Table of Contents

Preface

I was a chubby kid. These days, of course, a kid the same size would be labeled as obese, his parents told to starve him and run him lean for the sake of his health. But back then, I was just chubby or sometimes fat. Not that it made it any easier, being chubby instead of obese. The kids still picked on me. And when it came time for the dreaded annual one-mile run in gym class, I was always last—what seemed like hours behind everyone else.

When I was around the age of eleven, I had finally had enough of the teasing and taunting. Having also developed breasts, which felt shameful to me as a boy, I decided to remedy the whole situation by starving myself. Over the course of a summer, I ate practically nothing. I did all the usual kid stuff, including several weeks at Boy Scout camp, and with all the hormones of youth raging, I dropped pounds quickly.

As a child, I took piano lessons from a fat woman. Even her fingers were fat; she had to turn them sideways in order to avoid pressing two keys at the same time, though her fatness didn't prevent her from being a remarkably talented piano player.

Following that summer when I had begun starving myself, during one of my weekly piano lessons, my teacher turned to me with a look in her eyes that I'll never forget. She asked me, "How did you lose all the weight?" The look in her eyes was one of deep pain. She truly wanted to know my secret. I could see how much all the looks, the stares, the jokes at her expense, and the self-righteous comments she must have endured because of her size and shape must have hurt her.

Something happened to me in that moment. The relative carefree nature of youth vanished as I discovered that others could feel pain—perhaps even more deeply than I could.

But I couldn't tell her my secret. Despite the fact that it had been successful, I knew, as an animal must surely know without having to be told, that starving oneself is wrong. There is a biological imperative that must be overridden in order to successfully starve oneself. Even though some of us are able to do it, deep in our psyches we know it is antithetical to life. I couldn't bring myself to suggest that she starve herself. I had known this woman for more than half a decade, and in a strange way, I loved her. I couldn't inflict harm on someone I love. So I shrugged and said, "I dunno." And that was that.

For the next 20 years, I continued to starve myself. I restricted in one way or another. My weight remained low. Then lower. Then lower, until I looked like a skeleton and felt like one too. And over the years, the obsession with "health" grew until it was all consuming. The anxiety that I experienced initially was all about food and body image, but eventually became pervasive, overtaking all aspects of life.

Finally, gratefully, I was graced with the good fortune to begin eating again—something that, unfortunately, never happens for a great many people with long-term restrictive eating disorders. Fat, sugar, refined foods, carbohydrates—the stuff that had been off-limits was welcomed back onto my plate. Believe it or not, it was hard work to eat after all those years of not eating enough, but after a while the weight started to come back on and *I felt much better.*

As a result, I have a perspective on the whole so-called "obesity epidemic" that differs from most of the self-proclaimed experts. I've experienced the body shaming and humiliation that go along with being "overweight" and from having a body shape that is different from the accepted standard. But I have also experienced the horrors of overexercise and undernutrition.

Subsequently, I've done a lot of research into these matters—weight, weight loss, weight gain, body shape, appetite, metabolism, starvation, overfeeding, cardiovascular disease, diabetes, and so on. And while I can't say that I have the definitive answers, I can say that I've found that the conventional answers are dissatisfying and that there are a good many questions that should be asked but aren't being asked. That's what this book is about.

In all those years of piano lessons, I never saw my teacher eat anything more than tiny bowls of oatmeal. Was she secretly binging on Ho Hos at night? Sure, that's possible. But what if the stereotypes are wrong? What if much of what we think we know about fatness and health isn't the truth?

I've read story after story of fat people who eat fewer than 1000 calories a day and cannot lose weight. Their doctors call them liars. And we, the public, are allowed to judge them with impunity. We've been told that fat people are a burden to society. But what if we're not right? What if we're just cruel?

This book is an attempt to demonstrate that the story we believe is just a narrow piece of a bigger picture, and even much of that narrow piece is misleading or exaggerated. What follows is my humble attempt to invite us all to begin to take a look at ourselves, our fellow humans, and our cultures in a different light.

Am I biased? Yes. I believe that people have the right to dignity and kindness without consideration for their size or shape, whether they eat brown rice or Big Macs, and no matter how long they can run on a treadmill. I believe that the so-called "obesity epidemic" is little more than sanctioned scapegoating of innocent individuals. I believe that starvation is counterproductive to health and that most of the "health" advice these days (calorie restriction and overexercise) results in starvation. And I believe that we can do better.

However, despite my bias, I have attempted to present the following material fairly and without jumping to conclusions. So don't expect a lot of drama and intrigue in what follows. Instead, I try to present you with "just the facts" so that you can make up your own mind. Or, better yet, don't make up your own mind. Just open it instead.

Epidemic

Anyone who listens to the radio, browses a bookstore, or has a conversation with another human these days is likely reminded on a regular if not daily basis of the so-called "obesity epidemic"[1] said to be sweeping the globe. According to the Harvard School of Public Health and the World Health Organization (WHO), human waistlines are ballooning around the globe; the rates of clinical obesity *doubled* between 1980 and 2007, and by that year, 500 *million* adults across the globe were *dangerously* fat. Not just in the rich countries, but also in poorer places.

Many people who seem very important, very intelligent, and very sincere are hard at work trying to figure out why we're all so fat and what to do about it. So it's easy to get swept up in the drama and accept it all at face value. But there's a very important question that rarely gets asked: is fatness really a problem?

For many, the question doesn't even need to be asked because they already know the answer; fatness is a problem because it causes numerous preventable deaths. In fact, Julie Gerberding, then the director of the Centers for Disease Control (CDC),

---

[1] Technically, an epidemic is a widespread occurrence of an *infectious* disease. There is no reason to believe that fatness is contagious. So the use of the term "epidemic" is incorrect.

suggested a decade ago that in the United States alone 400,000[2] people were dying of fatness! Not only that, but we are also told that the health care costs associated with fatness are taking their toll on the taxpayers' bank accounts. In other words, fatness is a public burden.

Yet, as we'll see, in fact, people don't die because they are fat. The leading cause of death worldwide is cardiovascular disease. *That* is why people die, not fatness. For those who believe that cardiovascular disease is *caused* by fatness, this point may seem like splitting hairs. But as it turns out, there is no proof that being fat *causes* cardiovascular disease. And this is a very important point to understand. If cardiovascular disease is to blame, then the more honest view of the state of things is to speak of a "cardiovascular disease epidemic" rather than an "obesity epidemic."

Yet another question that rarely gets asked is whether the advice that is so commonplace—to lose weight—is actually good advice. Is the advice helping reduce the rates of disease and death? Can it?

In order to reduce the public burden and to save the poor, fat masses from their miserable fatness, huge efforts are being made to remind us of the importance of eating less and moving more. We're told that by exerting more willpower and trying harder, we can drop the pounds and stave off sickness. Over the decades, Weight Watchers, Ultra Slimfast, the pharmaceutical manufacturers of amphetamines and fen-phen (among many others), and bariatric surgeons—even liposuction surgeons— have all clambered to offer help to the "overweight." Because fatness is considered to be a major health risk, insurance companies will even cover some weight-loss procedures and drugs. But, as we'll see, despite the *billions* of dollars spent by individuals wishing to drop a few pounds (or a few dozen

---

[2] This figure later came under scrutiny, and the CDC backpedalled on the claim, but the number had already been etched into the public mind.

pounds…or a few hundred pounds), the rates of the diseases pinned on fatness are continuing to increase.

The more I learn, the clearer it becomes to me that blaming fatness for sickness is a view unsupported by scientific literature. And furthermore, blaming individuals for their fatness is generally unsupported by the literature as well. What I find is that all the talk about the so-called "obesity epidemic" is little more than thinly-veiled bigotry, the result of which is no reduction in disease while the majority of us are being shamed, humiliated, starved, and mutilated.

Throughout this book, I hope to take a fresh look at the situation. Although I don't propose to have all the answers or to have figured anything out, I do hope to call into question many of the firmly held assumptions that underpin what we might more fairly term the anti-fatness epidemic, or an epidemic of bigotry. Let's look together to see if perhaps there's more to the story than we've been told.

We're Getting Fatter All the Time

Many are quick to point out that there is much about the "obesity epidemic" that is overinflated—and not just waistlines. As we'll see, there are political and economic forces with a vested interest in the matter. And yet, as we'll also see, it would seem that we are, indeed, getting fatter.

To reinforce the *size* of the "epidemic," media outlets and health organizations alike frequently remind us of the statistics: of the 7.2 billion humans estimated to live on the planet, 11 percent are now classified as obese and 35 percent are classified as overweight. In the United States, one of the fattest nations, more than 35 percent of the adult population is classified as obese and over 68 percent are considered overweight.

On the surface, these numbers are staggering. But those with a more sober view remind us that it is easy to manipulate numbers to tell a story. And it turns out that is just what has happened. In 1997, the WHO published a paper titled "Obesity: preventing and managing the global epidemic" [3] in which new recommendations were made to define the terms "overweight" and "obesity" and set an international standard. The paper stirred up controversy and lots of questions among researchers and other professionals who knew a thing or two about fatness and

---

[3] World Health Organization. Report of a WHO consultation on obesity. Obesity: preventing and managing the global epidemic. Geneva: World Health Organization, 1998.

health. Why? Well, for a few reasons, not the least of which was that, among many, it was known that all-cause mortality (meaning how many people die from any cause) among those classified as overweight and "class I" obese by the new recommendations are actually *lower* than in the "normal" category.

The new WHO recommendations defined "normal" as a BMI (calculated as mass divided by the square of the height) of 18.5 to 24.9. From 25 to 29.9 became "overweight." And 30 and greater became "obese" with three classes of increasing obesity. Yet according to many researchers, positive correlations between BMI and all-cause mortality don't start to show up until the BMI is 35 or higher. Well, unless we consider any BMI *less* than 18.5, which correlates strongly with high rates of mortality!

The organization that led the charge in creating the recommendations and drafting the paper, the International Obesity Task Force (IOTF), received financial backing from pharmaceutical companies chomping at the bit to have a larger market for "weight-loss drugs." And according to a quote from Philip James (the chairman of the organization) that appeared in the UK newspaper, *The Guardian*, the charge is true, but he claims that the money came with no strings attached. He made the decisions he made because he felt it was the right thing to do.

In the WHO paper's acknowledgments, right after thanking James and the IOTF, there appears a note of gratitude to Xavier Pi-Sunyer of St. Luke's Roosevelt Hospital Center and Columbia University for his contributions. Yet when mentioning his affiliations, they failed to mention that he was also chairing the board of the Weight Watchers Foundation. (And yes, in case you were wondering, Weight Watchers Foundation is a subsidiary of Weight Watchers International—*that* Weight Watchers.)

In 1998, a National Institutes of Health commission headed by Xavier Pi-Sunyer (the same Xavier Pi-Sunyer, in case you were in doubt) chose to follow suit and utilize the same BMI categories as the WHO in order to define overweight and obesity. The NIH had previously defined "overweight" as BMI 27.8 or greater, but with the new definition, approximately 30 million American's were reclassified as overweight overnight.

Then there's the matter of using BMI as an indicator of body composition. Organizations such as the Center for Consumer Freedom, which is a food industry association with an obvious bias and conflict of interest, call into question whether BMI is of *any* value as an indicator of body composition when they point out that, based strictly on BMI, Sylvester Stallone, Arnold Schwarzenegger, Tom Cruise, Mel Gibson, Sammy Sosa, and The Rock are all obese while Michael Jordan, Pierce Brosnan, Brad Pitt, and George W. Bush are all overweight.

It is true that BMI does not actually indicate body composition (as it is calculated using height and weight alone). And it is also true that some of the early proponents of BMI specifically warned against using it as a way to diagnose the health of an individual. However, it is disingenuous to try to use the dismissal of the relevance of BMI as a way to dismiss the increasing prevalence of fatness by proxy. Why? Because without placing any spin on it, just by looking at the raw numbers, we do seem to be getting fatter.

Every year, the US National Center for Health Statistics conducts a national survey called the National Health and Nutrition Examination Survey (NHANES), which is an enormous collection of data that is publicly available for anyone who wishes to review it. Some of the data is self-reported, but a large amount of the data, including BMI reports, is measured. So it is reasonable to assume that height, weight, waist circumference, and skinfold measurements are reliable.

What does NHANES reveal? Well, at least in the United States, the average BMI has trended upward since the inception of the survey (1971), with the most pronounced increase beginning after 1980. Rates of "overweight" have remained fairly steady, but rates of "obesity" have increased nearly four-fold among men and nearly two-fold among women. Of course, as many critics have pointed out, BMI is not a perfect indicator of fatness. But, it turns out, the correlation is good enough. In fact, it turns out that BMI actually *under*estimates the amount of body fat for BMIs greater than 25. In other words, while BMI values indicate that we are getting fatter, measurements of body composition reveal that we're even fatter than BMI suggests!

While some analyses of the data suggest that certain racial or economic groups are more or less affected by the "epidemic," a more honest look at the data shows that all BMIs are rising among all groups. So all in all, it does seem that, relatively speaking, we are *all* getting fatter equally. It doesn't matter what our race, where we live, or how much money we have in the bank; the trends are all running parallel. As Thornton Melon might say, we've "ballooned up nicely."

In summary, we *do* appear to be getting fatter. At least in the U.S. that is the trend, and if we believe the numbers reported by the WHO, then similar trends are to be seen globally (with the exception of sub-Saharan Africa). If we are to believe the hype, then this evidence seems to confirm that there may well be an "epidemic" at hand. But rather than believing the hype, let's look to see if there is any evidence. Is fatness actually a problem in and of itself? In the next section, we'll look at this question.

In Fatness and Health

Although the leading voices prefer to use the term "obesity," I do not. I believe it is much more appropriate to use the term 'fatness' or other derivations. And the reason is simple: obesity is often defined as a *medical* condition, and any talk about obesity inherently frames the conversation such that we imagine that anyone who is fat must also be sick. Worse than that, we are often meant to imagine that fat people are a burden on society. And so to speak of an "obesity epidemic" is leading because the phrase itself suggests that there is a problem inherent in fatness.

However, surely the notion "innocent until proven guilty" should apply here. Until we know that fatness is *actually* a problem and *actually* the cause of sickness, it seems more appropriate to use a more neutral term such as fatness. (We could use the term "adiposity" to steer clear of the cultural derision often attached to the term "fat," but "adiposity" also lends itself to medicalization. So I'll just stick with "fatness.")

Fat is a substance. We all have it. In fact, we need it. Adipose tissue, which is what we usually think of when we speak of fat, serves many purposes, including insulation, organ protection, and energy supply. There is nothing intrinsically wrong with fat. And, in fact, there are a variety of cultures that *value* fatness on the human body. Many actually see fatness as a sign of health. So even the notion that fatness is inherently repulsive is untenable. Rather than jumping to conclusions and starting an investigation with preconceptions, it may be more fruitful for us to set aside prejudices for or against fatness and admit that until we can prove otherwise, fat is simply fat, and the meanings that are often attached to it are cultural, not strictly biological.

Of course, too much of a good thing isn't always a good thing. And too much of a neutral thing isn't always neutral. So just because *some* fat is necessary and healthy doesn't mean that more is always better. But let's take a look and see if fatness is inherently problematic.

For years we've been told that being fat *causes* sickness. In particular, we've been told that fatness causes cardiovascular disease and type 2 diabetes. But these claims are misleading on two accounts.

First, we simply do not know that fatness does *causes* sickness. Rather, there is a *correlation* between sickness and BMI. As BMI rises above 35, there is a clear increase in deaths. (Note that 35 is well above 25, which is now the upper limit for what is considered healthy.) But here we are best to remember what researchers often remind us: correlation does not mean causation. Just because people with higher BMIs have higher incidences of some diseases does not mean that fatness causes the diseases. It's also worth mentioning that the association between BMI and death rates is relatively weak in those under age 50. The association becomes much stronger for those over the age of 50 and gets stronger with each decade after 50. But one is left to wonder at the fact that, completely independent of BMI, it would seem that *advanced age* is the greatest risk factor for death, a matter we'll explore in more detail shortly.

Secondly, the suggestion that a BMI greater than 25 (which is how overweight is defined now) is a problem completely misrepresents that actual data. In a paper published in the *International Journal of Obesity*,[4] the authors show that mortality rates graphed by BMI reveal a U-shaped curve where mortality

---

[4] Douglas K. Childers, PhD and David B. Allison, PhD, "The 'Obesity Paradox:' a parsimonious explanation for relations among obesity, mortality rate, and aging?," *International Journal of Obesity* (August 2010): 1231-1238.

rates increased most markedly with *low* BMI and more moderately with high BMI. The lowest mortality rates tend to be in the 20-35 range, and higher BMI is correlated with lower mortality rates as age increases (though rates of mortality still increase rapidly above BMI 35). But the greatest rise in mortality is for BMIs *below* 20.

In a paper published in the *Journal of the American Medical Association*,[5] the authors performed a meta-analysis of 97 studies involving 2.88 million people. What they found was that people with a BMI between 25 and 35 had fewer deaths than those with a BMI between 18.5 and 25, which is normally considered healthy.

Doctors and public health professionals (not to mention diet book authors, personal trainers, weight-loss companies, bariatric surgeons, and pharmaceutical companies) around the world seem to have become obsessed with "helping" fat people to become thin all in the name of health. But when one looks at the data and *particularly* when one remembers that correlation does not equal causation, this zeal to convert the fat masses to skinny minnies starts to seem a bit...misguided.

Oftentimes we are told that losing weight will reduce risk for some diseases. Yet it turns out that it's just not that simple. Although the correlation between high BMI and death rates exists for anyone to see, no one yet knows what, if anything, that correlation signifies. And the more that researchers study the matter, the more they are uncovering the nuances that demonstrate that fatness is not inherently problematic. Take, for example, a study conducted by the Massachusetts General Hospital,[6] which found that many people who are classified as

---

[5] Flegal, K. M., Kit, B. K., Orpana, H. & Graubard, B. I., "Association of All-Cause Mortality With Overweight and Obesity Using Standard Body Mass Index Categories," *Journal of the American Medical Association* 309 (January 2013): 71–82.

[6] Meigs et al., "Body Mass Index, Metabolic Syndrome, and Risk of Type 2 Diabetes or Cardiovascular Disease," *Journal of Clinical Endocrinology and Metabolism* (August 2006): 2906-2912.

obese have no actual increased risk of disease while many who are normal weight have increased risk of the very diseases that are normally considered to be the result of fatness! Or consider the so-called "obesity paradox,"[7] which is a puzzle that has many people scratching their heads; people classified as overweight and obese often have better rates of survival than their skinnier counterparts when it comes to a variety of diseases such as heart disease, heart failure, peripheral arterial disease, stroke, osteoporosis, and diabetes[8] to name a few. One has to wonder if everyone is barking up the wrong fat tree. Maybe fatness in and of itself isn't a problem. Or, at least, maybe it's not always or even mostly a problem.

It is interesting that despite all the hype about weight loss, it turns out that for those who already have diseases, losing weight doesn't necessarily offer any benefits. A study supported by the National Institutes of Health called the Look AHEAD study[9] was a ten-year study that began with 5145 people, hoping to demonstrate that weight loss would significantly improve health for diabetics, and this study actually demonstrated *no improvement*. The intervention group was placed on a *severely* restricted diet with a maximum of 1800 calories a day and with some restricted to as little as 1000 calories a day until they lost between 7 and 10 percent of body weight. This was done in the first year. They were also required to do at least 175 minutes of moderate-intensity exercise each week, and this was to be maintained for the next several years. From the fifth year onward, the researchers reviewed the outcomes for the participants.

---

[7] Hainer, V. and Aldhoon-Hainerova, I., "Obesity Paradox Does Exist," *Diabetes Care* (August 2013): S276-281.

[8] The "obesity paradox" in regard to diabetes has been contested by a study; Tobias et al., "Body-mass index and mortality among adults with incident type 2 diabetes.," *New England Journal of Medicine* (January 2014): 233-244.

[9] The Look AHEAD Research Group, "Cardiovascular Effects of Intensive Lifestyle Intervention in Type 2 Diabetes," *New England Journal of Medicine* (July 2013): 145-154.

Of the 5145 original participants, only 1193 completed the study. Given that the calorie allowances were within the ranges that have previously been shown to produce states of semi-starvation in the monumental Minnesota Starvation Experiment, it is no surprise that so many participants would have dropped out: semi-starvation is known to produce a long list of very unpleasant and potentially life-threatening symptoms.

So what did the researchers in the Look AHEAD study find? They found that the intervention group, despite maintaining a 6 percent weight loss after ten years, showed no significant reduction in heart attacks, strokes, or angina over the control group. Granted, the intervention group did show some improvements such as better glycemic control and less sleep apnea, but it is impossible to tell whether these results were because of weight loss or because of the nature of the intervention. For example, the Look AHEAD document states that "[t]he composition of the diet is structured to enhance glycemic control." Given that the diet composition was designed to enhance glycemic control, it isn't a surprise to see an improvement in glycemic control as a result. But that doesn't mean it has anything to do with weight loss. And moderate increases in physical activity—completely independent of weight loss—are often associated with improvements in health. So the Look AHEAD study lends some support to the notion that weight isn't likely a major determinant to health. Rather, other factors probably play a much more important role. Perhaps genetics and other environmental factors are much more important than weight.

What seems to be the case is that there are studies that demonstrate that particular interventions (e.g., a diet composition designed to enhance glycemic control) may sometimes offer health benefits when applied appropriately and for the right people (e.g., diabetics probably benefit from diets that offer improved glycemic control whereas non-diabetics may not). When studies are not specifically looking at weight, the results tend to be clearer. For example, a paper published in the *Journal of the American Medical Association* in 2004 [10] concluded that adhering to the Mediterranean Diet, moderate (as opposed to high) alcohol use, physical activity, and non-smoking all correlated with significant decreases in mortality rates. But these factors are independent of weight or fatness.

What is becoming increasingly clear to me the more that I research the matter is that, despite the hype, there simply isn't much evidence demonstrating that fatness is inherently a problem. Fatness is not necessarily an indicator of health problems. In fact, moderate fatness often correlates to good health whereas even moderately low fatness (meaning BMI less than 20) often correlates with poor health. Does this mean that fatness may not sometimes be indicative of poor health in *some* people? Of course not. Fatness, *in some cases*, may indicate an underlying health problem. However, that does not mean that fatness is *always* or even often a good indicator of poor health. And furthermore, it does not mean that losing weight in and of itself will fix any health problems that fatness may indicate.

The more I research, the more I suspect that all talk of fatness (or, rather "overweight" and "obesity," as it is usually described) is focusing on the wrong thing. Consider for a moment that paleness is a symptom often seen in cases of anemia, but it would be a mistake to confuse the symptom for the cause. After all, simply changing the appearance of the skin won't resolve anemia. And it may be that fixating on fatness and weight loss as a cure for disease is like trying to cure anemia by way of a spray-on tan. It may be misguided.

Since fatness hasn't yet been convicted of killing anyone, I'm going to err on the side of innocence until guilt is proven. Instead of focusing on fat, which may be nothing more than a sometimes-concurrent symptom of some diseases, might it be more productive to look at the *actual* causes of death and examine the

---

[10] Knoops, K.T., de Groot, L.C., Kromhout, D. et al., "Mediterranean diet, lifestyle factors, and 10-year mortality in elderly European men and women: the HALE project," *Journal of the American Medical Association* (2004): 1433–1439.

known and likely causes of those conditions—not just the symptoms such as fatness?

The two primary categories of disease that are often associated with fatness are type 2 diabetes and cardiovascular disease. In the sections that follow, we'll explore these diseases, including what is known about them, including known causes. We'll also explore some theories to see if there may be other factors (including environmental factors) that could contribute to the diseases that extend beyond simply blaming the individual for being fat, gluttonous, and lazy.

The Rise of Diabetes

Diabetes mellitus (more commonly just "diabetes") is a condition of impaired blood sugar control. Normally, this is a result of reduced (or non-existent) insulin production, insulin resistance, or both. Normally, the pancreas (a gland behind the stomach) produces a hormone called insulin, which, among other things, is thought to transport glucose (sugar) from the blood into muscles and organs. When insulin production is too low or when insulin resistance in muscles and most organs is too great, blood sugar may remain high, causing damage.

The pancreas has specialized cells called beta cells that produce insulin. In type 1 and type 2 diabetes, the most common types, beta cells become damaged. It is believed that in type 1 diabetes, beta cell damage is due to genetic or environmental factors, and this type of diabetes normally begins at a younger age when compared to type 2. Type 2 diabetes, however, accounts for 90% of diabetes cases worldwide. In type 2, beta cell damage may sometimes occur *prior to* or without insulin resistance. However, in other cases, insulin resistance may occur prior to detected beta cell damage. In either case, eventually the problem is caused by reduced insulin production due to beta cell damage.

If the onset of type 2 diabetes is preceded by insulin resistance, then it is possible that the person will experience fat gain. The reason for this may be that insulin resistance develops in muscles and many organs, but not in adipose tissue, which is actually an organ in its own right. It is believed that the reason that other parts of the body develop insulin resistance is because of impaired cellular respiration, and the resistance to insulin prevents too much glucose from entering a cell with impaired function and thus doing damage. Adipose tissue, on the other hand, can "mop up" glucose, turning it into fat, and preventing damage to the rest of the body. So far, it doesn't sound like fat is *causing* diabetes. Rather, it sounds as though increased fat storage *may* sometimes indicate insulin resistance, which *may* be indicative of an underlying problem.

In any case, diabetes is not a condition to which anyone should aspire. It comes with a whole bunch of possible complications, including heart problems, foot problems, eye problems, kidney problems, and more. And so if diabetes is in fact preventable, then it certainly is sensible to take reasonable steps to prevent the disease. And, if the prevalence of diabetes truly is increasing, that may be cause for concern if there is something that can be done about it. In this section, we'll look to see if diabetes is on the rise, and if it is, we'll look to see if it might be preventable.

According to NHANES III (1988-1994), the percentage of Americans with a fasting glucose level above 126 mg/l (indicating possible diabetes[11]) was 7.5. I ran the numbers using the 2010 NHANES data and found that the percentage had increased to 9.6. And just to be sure it wasn't a fluke, I also looked at the intervening years and found that there did, in fact, seem to be an upward trend.

The CDC reports new cases of type 2 diabetes diagnosed by year in the U.S. from 1980 to 2009, but doesn't cite the source of the data. Furthermore, since the CDC data is for new diagnoses, it doesn't necessarily give a very clear picture of how many people have severely impaired glucose tolerance whereas the NHANES data does. However, the CDC data is useful because it gives at least some idea of trends over time, and what it shows is that from 1980 to the early 90s, the rates of new diagnoses was fairly

---

[11] Diabetes is diagnosed by measuring plasma glucose, but high blood sugar may or may not be the result of beta cell damage.

constant, but in the early 90s a dramatic upturn began, and by the year 2009 the number of new annual diagnoses had quadrupled. Something seems to be happening.

In 1997, the American Diabetes Association and the U.S. government redefined how type 2 diabetes is diagnosed. Whereas the old standard was a fasting glucose of 140 mg/l or greater, the new cut-off became 126 mg/l. The effect, one would suspect, would be a dramatic increase in the number of diagnoses. However, according to the CDC data, the trend began well before 1997 and continued steadily afterward.

The International Diabetes Federation (IDF) claims that 382 million people worldwide have diabetes (the vast majority of which have type 2 diabetes) as of 2014, and that the number is expected to rise to 592 million by the year 2035. To put those numbers in perspective, that's 5.3 percent of the world population at present, and 6.8 percent by 2035 (since dramatic population increases are expected over the next several decades). So the IDF predictions seem to be in line with the increases reported in the U.S. over the past few decades, according to NHANES.

Thus, it does seem that no matter which way we look at it, there is an increase in cases of diabetes. But the question begs to be asked, *why*? And *that* is the $64,000 question. Why indeed?

When I started investigating diabetes trends, I noticed something interesting, though not particularly surprising: rates of diabetes increase with age. In other words, one of the greatest risk factors for diabetes is increased age.[12] So out of curiosity, I investigated to see what the trends in population aging are. Once again, not surprisingly, worldwide population is aging significantly. According to a United Nations report, [13] the

---

[12] These trends are visible in the NHANES data. Diabetes diagnoses are low until age 45, then increase dramatically with each decade until age 75 when the number drops back to 55-64 levels. Presumably that is because after age 75 many cases of diabetes have been diagnosed.

[13] World Population Ageing 2013

worldwide share of people over the age of 60 increased from 9.2 percent in 1990 to 11.7 percent in 2013 "and will continue to grow as a proportion of the world population, reaching 21.1 percent by 2050." And the United Nations Population Fund website shows that this trend has been happening since at least 1960.

Is it possible that the increasing rates of diabetes can be explained away solely by an increasingly aging population? While possible, it seems unlikely, but it certainly suggests a possibility that the scale of the "epidemic" is often overstated. This is borne out by the fact that according to the CDC[14] using data from the National Health Interview Survey, the most significant increases in diagnoses of diabetes over the past several decades are seen in populations over the age of 45. There are some very modest increases in diagnoses among those under the age of 45, but the significance of this is hard to determine. For one thing, screening for diabetes has become much more aggressive in recent decades, and so it is possible that that fact alone may account for the increases in diagnoses among younger people.

Obviously, short of a developing a time machine, age is not a preventable risk factor. But, of course, it's not the only risk factor. Some other major risk factors include genetics and ethnicity, and like age, there's nothing we can do about these factors. Being poor is another major risk factor,[15] but winning the lottery doesn't seem to help. And those who never completed high school education are also at greater risk,[16] but getting a GED doesn't seem to mitigate the risk.

Now, you may think I'm being flip by pointing out all the risk factors that clearly aren't causative such as socioeconomic class

---

[14] http://www.cdc.gov/diabetes/statistics/incidence/fig3.htm

[15] Chih-Cheng et al., "Poverty Increases Type 2 Diabetes Incidence and Inequality of Care Despite Universal Health Coverage," *Diabetes Care* (November 2012): 2286-2292.

[16] Saydah, S.S .and Lochner, K., "Socioeconomic Status and Risk of Diabetes-Related Mortality in the U.S.," *Public Health Reports* (May-June 2010): 377-388.

and educational level, but that's not my intention. Rather, I merely intend to point out that *correlation does not equal causation*. So just as winning a bunch of money on Wheel of Fortune doesn't suddenly reduce risk, losing a bunch of fat doesn't necessarily reduce risk either, in and of itself.

It occurred to me that in order to determine whether fat loss alone can produce beneficial metabolic changes that actually reduce risk of developing diabetes, it would be necessary to have a procedure that allows for fat loss independent of lifestyle changes. And it turns out that such a procedure exists: liposuction. Not surprisingly, I'm not the only one that thought of this. Turns out that the U.S. government has funded some studies to find out whether liposuction can actually reduce the risk of diabetes. In 2001, a pilot study was published in *Plastic and Reconstructive Surgery* [17] in which the researchers selected 14 "overweight" women (with a mean BMI of 28.8, which, as we've already seen, actually is anything *but* overweight for many, if not most women) and removed an average of 5.1 kg of fat from each. They took a bunch of readings on the women before and after and concluded that liposuction may reduce risk for disease such as diabetes.

Well, not so fast. According to the report, liposuction did not affect cholesterol levels, triglycerides, or metabolic rate. And while they did measure a reduction in fasting insulin, the actual change and the causes of that change aren't clear. For one thing, in addition to the 5.1 kg of fat removed by liposuction, the women also lost another 1.3 kg over the next 6-8 weeks following the procedure. The experiment was not controlled at all. And it is quite possible that the effects seen in the experiment, as are often the case in these sorts of experiments, are due to the participants *wanting* to lose weight. Perhaps the liposuction provided the impetus for the women to make other changes that

---

[17] Giese et al., "Improvements in cardiovascular risk profile with large-volume liposuction: a pilot study," *Plastic and Reconstructive Surgery* (August 2001): 510-519.

could account for both further weight loss and a reduction in fasting insulin.

In any case, subsequent investigations into whether or not liposuction can reduce diabetes risk, including those published in more *reputable* publications such as the *New England Journal of Medicine*,[18] have concluded that liposuction does not provide any long-term risk reduction for diabetes or cardiovascular disease.

On the other hand, many studies show that when people who are considered to be at risk for developing diabetes lose weight, the risk of actually developing diabetes decreases significantly. For example, a paper published in *Diabetes Care* in 2006 [19] followed up with over 1000 participants over 3.2 years and found that those who lost weight *through lifestyle intervention* had much lower incidences of diabetes. And a longer-term study[20] showed that in ten years, weight loss correlated with much lower rates of diabetes while weight gain correlated with much higher rates.

But then the question is, does weight loss or weight gain *cause* fewer or greater incidences of diabetes? Or is it simply that those who are likely to develop diabetes are also likely to gain weight while those who aren't likely to develop diabetes may lose weight more easily? This is a question for which we may not yet have enough information to answer, so I pose it here as something that it may do us all well to consider before we jump to convenient conclusions and assume that those who have diabetes deserve it for not working harder to lose weight and prevent their illness. Though that sentiment is popular, it is not a fair or accurate assessment of the known information.

---

[18] Klein et al., "Absence of an effect of liposuction on insulin action and risk factors for coronary heart disease.," *New England Journal of Medicine* (June 2004): 2549-2557.

[19] Hamman et al., "Effect of weight loss with lifestyle intervention on risk of diabetes." *Diabetes Care* (September 2006): 2012-2017.

[20] Resnick et al., "Relation of weight gain and weight loss on subsequent diabetes risk in overweight adults," *Journal of Epidemiology and Community Health* (August 2000): 596-602.

Given that liposuction does not seem to result in risk reduction, it seems unlikely that fat loss alone can significantly reduce the incidences of diabetes. Yet there is some evidence that weight loss through lifestyle intervention seems to reduce the risk. As such, it seems logical that *if* a lifestyle intervention can actually reduce the risk, then it is the intervention itself that reduces the risk and weight loss is perhaps a side effect. [21] However, as I've already pointed out, we don't know whether the interventions (calorie restriction, macronutrient changes, increased physical activity) themselves actually produce the reduction in risk or if they merely reveal where underlying factors are likely to result in diabetes (indicated by the inability of an individual to lose weight or the regain of the weight, for example).

All in all, there's a lot more study needed before anyone can claim with certainty that specific lifestyle changes can actually produce any real change.

---

[21] It is also possible, of course, to explain this by way of the placebo effect since those who lose weight cannot be made blind to that fact, and the notion that losing weight will improve health is etched into most of our minds.

The Rise of Heart Disease

Now that we've looked at diabetes, let's get an overview of cardiovascular disease. Cardiovascular disease is an umbrella term for conditions related to the heart and/or blood vessels and includes things such as coronary heart disease (which may result in a heart attack), stroke, hypertension (high blood pressure), and heart failure.

According to the CDC and the WHO, cardiovascular disease remains the leading cause of death in the U.S. and worldwide, respectively. And, like diabetes, many of the major risk factors for cardiovascular disease are immutable. In fact, the risk factors for cardiovascular disease are very similar to those of diabetes. Age may be one of the most significant, as are ethnicity and genetics. And, like diabetes, poverty and a lack of a completed high school education are risk factors. But, you guessed it, working overtime and studying hard won't improve the situation. (In fact, the resultant lack of sleep might worsen things!) Men are more likely to develop cardiovascular disease, but a sex change operation probably won't reduce the risk (though no one has tested that hypothesis yet).

In the United States and in other so-called "developed" countries, the rates of death from cardiovascular disease are on the decline, presumably because of more aggressive treatment options and the money to implement them. While they may be on the decline, they are still high and still the single most significant category for cause of death. Furthermore, the indication is that the prevalence of cardiovascular disease, particularly coronary heart disease, is still either on the rise or has leveled out in the United States. And worldwide the rates of death are continuing to increase.[22]

So cardiovascular disease is kind of a big deal. But as we've already seen, some of the major risk factors aren't modifiable, which leaves us with the identified and popular risk factors that *are* modifiable, including fatness, smoking, and excessive alcohol consumption. Of these, the one that we're concerned with in this book is fatness, and, like diabetes, it's hard to say that fatness *causes* cardiovascular disease. Instead, it could be that cardiovascular disease and fatness may sometimes have a common cause.

As we saw earlier, liposuction probably doesn't reduce the incidence of diabetes. Neither does it likely reduce the incidence of cardiovascular disease or cardiovascular events. So it seems that fat loss alone probably isn't an effective way to improve one's health.

Multiple human trials have demonstrated that weight loss often improves *markers* for cardiovascular risk, but just because the values of some tests show up within a particular range doesn't necessarily mean anything about real-world occurrences. The question is, does weight loss correlate positively with reduced cardiovascular disease events? Surprisingly, very few studies have been done to attempt to answer this. However, one Israeli study published in 2005[23] followed up with 1,669 participants (age 50-75) for four years after they underwent six months of nutritional counseling and a weight-loss diet. The researchers found that those who maintained a weight loss had a significant reduction in

[22] Cannon, B., "Cardiovascular disease: Biochemistry to behavior," *Nature* (January 2013) S2-S3.

[23] Eilat-Adar et al., "Association of Intentional Changes in Body Weight with Coronary Heart Disease Event Rates in Overweight Subjects Who Have an Additional Coronary Risk Factor," *American Journal of Epidemiology* (2005): 352-358.

cardiovascular disease events when compared to those who did not lose or maintain a lower weight.

Much like our investigation of diabetes, here it seems that fat loss alone may not improve cardiovascular risk, but sustained weight loss seems to be a predictor of reduced risk. Why might that be so? If it's not the fat, per se, then we should consider other factors. For example, if someone is capable of losing weight and maintaining weight loss, that may be an indicator of several things, including the possibility that the person is in good health. We simply don't know what it is about sustained weight loss that might make it a predictor of reduced risk.

Low-Fat Donuts

N ow that we've gotten an overview of the situation regarding both diabetes and cardiovascular disease, we've started to see that fatness in and of itself may not matter. Yet, on the other hand, the act of losing weight and maintaining a lower weight *may* reduce risk for some people. So whether or not the weight loss itself is significant, it seems that the *way* in which people lose weight (or not) *may* be useful in reducing risk. In general, whether one is told to make lifestyle changes to reduce diabetes risk or cardiovascular risk, the advice is very similar: eat less fat (especially saturated fat), eat less sugar, eat less of everything (calorie restriction), and move more. In these next few sections, we'll look at each of these recommendations to see what the research suggests may or may not be effective for truly reducing risk.

First, we'll look at the standard advice regarding dietary fat. Whether the advice is coming from the American Diabetic Association (ADA), the American Heart Association (AHA), the CDC, the WHO, the IDF, or just about any other mainstream source, when it comes to dietary fat, the recommendation is to eat less. But *in particular*, we are told to eat *much less* saturated fat than we would otherwise do and instead, if we must eat fat (and most of us must, being the gluttonous sort who lack the necessary willpower to "succeed" in the war against fat), then we are told to eat "heart healthy" vegetable oils. No, not tropical oils that come from plants such as coconut or palm, since those contain "dangerous" saturated fats. Instead, we are told to eat canola, soy, corn, and safflower oil, which while known as "vegetable" oils, are more appropriately called industrial *seed* oils (because industrial processes are needed to separate the oil fractions from the plant material and they all come from the seeds of the respective plants).

According to the USDA (U.S. Department of Agriculture), the production of vegetable oils worldwide has increased rather dramatically over the past century. In particular, soy oil and corn oil were extremely rare a century ago, and canola oil didn't even exist until the 1970s. How much of an increase are we talking about? Take soy oil, for example. In a paper published in the *American Journal of Clinical Nutrition*,[24] the authors tell us that between 1909 and 1999 the consumption of soy oil as a food in the United States increased more than 1000 fold!

Regarding canola—an extremely popular "heart healthy" oil that even has a qualified health claim that has been approved by the Food and Drug Administration[25]—as noted, this oil didn't even exist until the 1970s. Canola is produced from the seed of a cruciferous plant called rapeseed. Rapeseed has been in use as a fuel for a long time, but it was never suitable for use in large amounts in food because of the toxic substance that it contains called erucic acid. However, in the 1970s, two agricultural scientists in Canada bred a low-erucic acid variety that was deemed suitable for food use.

In 1985, the U.S. FDA approved canola oil for use in food, and thus began the rapid rise of canola oil, particularly in the U.S., which is now the largest consumer of canola oil in the world.

---

[24] Blasbalg et al., "Changes in consumption of omega-3 and omega-6 fatty acids in the United States during the 20th century," *American Journal of Clinical Nutrition* (May 2011): 950-962.

[25]

http://www.fda.gov/food/ingredientspackaginglabeling/labelingnutrition/ucm072958.htm

According to the USDA,[26] the U.S. consumption of canola oil has steadily increased from next to nothing in 1985 to over 2.8 *billion* pounds in 2008 and 2009. And, according to the same source, most of that is used for food. And worldwide the demand keeps on growing, with the USDA estimating that between 2002 and 2011, worldwide production has nearly *quadrupled*.

So the first thing we might take away from this is that people are eating more polyunsaturated fat than ever before. And that seems to be the case. Furthermore, according to the NHANES data as shown in Figure 1,[27] since 1971, Americans are eating less saturated fat and less total fat. In other words, it would seem that at least in the U.S., people are taking the advice "to heart" (sorry for the terrible pun).

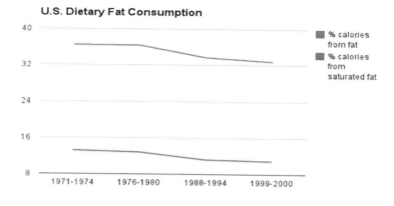

Figure 1

---

[26] http://www.ers.usda.gov/topics/crops/soybeans-oil-crops/canola.aspx

[27] It is important to note that the NHANES diet data is self-reported, and there is good reason to believe that the data isn't terrifically reliable. For example, many people underreport the number of calories that they eat in a day in most surveys when compared to studies in which actual calorie intake is monitored. And self-reports may be influenced by the current social values (i.e., reducing dietary fat intake is "good"). Therefore, we cannot know for certain how reliable this data is, but it does give some indicator as to possible trends.

But wait a second! As we've already seen, both diabetes and cardiovascular disease are on the rise in the U.S. and worldwide. If eating less fat and replacing saturated fat with polyunsaturated fat is supposed to reduce risk, then something seems amiss. And, in fact, it would seem that what we have here are the makings of a null hypothesis, meaning that the data doesn't support the theory.

Still, there are those who claim that the fact that Americans and others are complying with the guidelines is the reason why there are fewer *deaths* attributed to these diseases and why cholesterol levels have dropped over the years.[28] But while we cannot deny that as a possibility, it seems disingenuous to suggest it as a *probability* since rates of diabetes and cardiovascular disease have continued to *increase*.

So, on the surface, it would seem that eating less fat and replacing saturated fat (as is found in animal fats, butter, and tropical oils) with vegetable oils hasn't actually reduced the risk of diabetes or cardiovascular disease. But let's allow for the possibility that the data is misleading; maybe eating less saturated fat and less fat in general really *should* be a good idea. Yet one has to wonder, where did the idea come from? And has it been tested in ways other than epidemiological studies that tend to disprove the theory?

When I was doing research for my book *Food Myths*, I wanted to find out if there was any good evidence linking fat (particularly saturated fat) to cardiovascular disease or type 2 diabetes. What I found was surprising.

It turns out that the primary driver for the (saturated) fat phobia that is so prevalent today can be traced back to the work of Ancel Keys, the very same brilliant researcher who led the Minnesota Starvation Experiment. His brilliance is hard to dispute, but it seems fairly clear now that in some of his

---

[28] Dixon, .LB. and Ernst, N.D., "Choose a Diet That Is Low in Saturated Fat and Cholesterol and Moderate in Total Fat: Subtle Changes to a Familiar Message," *Journal of Nutrition* (February 2001): 5105-5265.

epidemiological work, he drew at least one wrong conclusion when he insisted that high fat intake, particularly saturated fat, led to increased risk of cardiovascular disease. In fact, it would seem that opposition to his conclusions was substantial early on in large part because they defied logic; numerous traditional cultures around the world have lived and continue to live in a virtual absence of cardiovascular disease and diabetes while eating large amounts of saturated fat. Many laughed at his theory, and some took the time to refute it. In 1957, two men named Yerushalmy and Hilleboe published a criticism of his theory. Here's an excerpt from *Food Myths* that explains the criticism.

Yerushalmy and Hilleboe point out that while countries with higher levels of saturated fat available have higher rates of reported cardiovascular disease, overall they have considerably lower rates of disease when compared to countries with lower levels of saturated fat available. They also point out that higher levels of saturated fat correlate with wealth in the data. And they go on to suggest that less wealthy countries were likely grossly under-reporting cardiovascular disease deaths, instead classifying them as something else.

The real wrench in the works, however, is that the data Keys was working from was simply a report of what food existed in a country. He wasn't looking at what people actually were eating. So at the end of the day, although Keys' graphs may be interesting, they didn't tell us anything about real world trends.

When Keys presented his findings to the WHO in 1955, he was met with much criticism. And despite his efforts to persuade major organizations such as the American Heart Association about the dangers of fat, particularly saturated fat, none listened to his pleas to recommend that the masses reduce fat intake. At least not at first. But finally, after Keys landed a spot on the board, the American Heart Association cracked and began to promote the idea that a diet high in animal fats and tropical fats caused cardiovascular disease. The idea gained traction, and in the late 1970s, the U.S government began to toe the line.

The only trouble is that there simply has never been any good evidence that the theory was correct. The few long-term, well-designed studies that have been conducted, such as the L.A.

Veteran's Trial, demonstrate no significant decrease in cardiovascular deaths among those placed on a low-saturated-fat diet versus control. And recent meta-analysis studies [29] , [30] conclude that there "is no significant evidence for concluding that dietary saturated fat is associated with an increased risk of CHD [stroke] or CVD [cardiovascular disease]" and "current evidence does not clearly support cardiovascular guidelines that encourage high consumption of polyunsaturated fatty acids and low consumption of total saturated fats." In fact, now the tides have turned so much that in June 2014, *Time* magazine ran a headline on the cover that said, "Eat Butter. Scientists labeled fat the enemy. Why they were wrong."

Not only are the standard recommendations to lower total fat and *especially* saturated fat unhelpful, they go the extra mile and recommend replacing saturated fats with "heart healthy" polyunsaturated fats, specifically recommending vegetable oils such as corn oil and soybean oil. But these oils are extremely high in omega-6 fatty acids, the type of fatty acids that are linked with increased inflammation.[31,32] Inflammation is a major contributor to both cardiovascular disease[33] *and* type 2 diabetes.[34]

Saturated fat—particularly naturally occurring saturated fat in animal fats and tropical oils—has gotten a bad rap not only in

---

[29] Chowdhury et al., "Association of Dietary, Circulating, and Supplement Fatty Acids With Coronary Risk," *Annals of Internal Medicine* (March 2014): 398-406.

[30] Siri-Tarino et al., "Meta-analysis of prospective cohort studies evaluating the association of saturated fat with cardiovascular disease," *American Journal of Clinical Nutrition* (March 2010): 535-546.

[31] Simopoulos, A.P., "Importance of the ratio of omega-6/omega-3 essential fatty acids: evolutionary aspects.," *World Review of Nutrition and Dietetics* (2003): 1-22.

[32] James et al., "Dietary polyunsaturated fatty acids and inflammatory mediator production," *The American Journal of Clinical Nutrition* (2000): 343-348.

[33] Libby, P., "Inflammation and cardiovascular disease mechanisms.," *American Journal of Clinical Nutrition* (February 2006): 456-460.

[34] Donath, M.Y., Shoelson, S.E., "Type 2 diabetes as an inflammatory disease.," *Nature Review. Immunology* (February 2011): 98-107.

regard to cardiovascular disease, but also in regard to insulin resistance. Some have attempted to link dietary saturated fat consumption with increased incidences of insulin resistance, but no one has been able to make the accusation stick. In a 2009 study published in the *American Journal of Clinical Nutrition*,[35] the authors concluded that humans eating a high-saturated-fat diet did not show any changes in insulin sensitivity. [36] And in a 2011 LIPGENE study, [37] the authors concluded that reducing saturated fat intake did not improve insulin sensitivity.

Finally, just for kicks, let's see if dietary fat contributes to fatness. For the past few decades, we've been told that it does, and low-fat foods have been marketed as diet foods that can help us to lose weight. But in the end, it turns out to make no difference. As Walter Willett, M.D., chair of the department of nutrition at Harvard School of Public Health (and an outspoken advocate of weight loss) writes in an article published in the *American Journal of Medicine*,[38] "Diets high in fat do not appear to be the primary cause of the high prevalence of excess body fat in our society, and reductions in fat will not be a solution."

---

[35] Van Dijk et al., "A saturated fatty acid-rich diet induces an obesity-linked proinflammatory gene expression profile in adipose tissue of subjects at risk of metabolic syndrome.," *American Journal of Clinical Nutrition* (December 2009): 1656-1664.

[36] The authors did suggest that a high-saturated fat diet may increase pro-inflammatory gene expression. However, other studies have shown that adequate omega-3 fatty acid intake offsets any inflammatory effects whereas the same is not true of high omega-6 polyunsaturated fat diets, which also exert pro-inflammatory effects but cannot be offset with omega-3 fatty acids.

[37] Tierney et al., "Effects of dietary fat modification on insulin sensitivity and on other risk factors of the metabolic syndrome—LIPGENE: a European randomized dietary intervention study.," *International Journal of Obesity* (June 2011): 800-809.

[38] Willett, W.C., Leibel ,R.L., "Dietary fat is not a major determinant of body fat," *American Journal of Medicine* (December 2013) Supplement 9B: 47-59.

Sugar-Free Donuts

For more than half a century, organizations such as the American Heart Association and the American Diabetes Association have been warning us about the dangers of saturated fat, cholesterol, salt, and other dietary evils, but there has been little to no warning about sugar. The AHA has only recently begun to give lip service to the idea that sugar may be a health problem, almost as if testing the waters before deciding whether to jump on the anti-sugar bandwagon. The ADA, on the other hand, still gives very little caution regarding dietary sugar beyond the sensible suggestion to limit sugary beverages.

As we'll see in this section, there is very little evidence linking dietary sugar—at least natural (non-industrial) sugar—to cardiovascular disease or the development of type 2 diabetes. But as we'll also see, there's a new wave of fanaticism that is sweeping the world, claiming that dietary sugar of all kinds, even carrots and potatoes, may be the cause of every ill known to humans. And as such, many of us now think that there is a proven causal link between dietary sugar (or carbohydrates in general) and disease as well as fatness.

It seems that every few decades the "health pundits" proclaim a new a dietary devil. Saturated fat was once to blame. Then salt. Then cholesterol. But as the old devils are exonerated (by science, though not by the establishment), new devils have to be made. In the last decade or so, sugar is the luciferian substance du jour. From "childhood obesity expert" Robert Lustig to journalist

Gary Taubes to low-carb diet gurus like Mark Sisson, we needn't look far to learn about the many supposed evils of sugar.

Once not that long ago, the word "sugar" in most conversations referred only to the white stuff Mom kept in a dish for spooning into coffee or maybe the brown stuff sprinkled atop oatmeal or baked into cookies. In other words, sucrose, with or without the molasses, made from sugar cane or sugar beets. But in recent years, the conversations have changed some, and even in casual conversations, "sugar" may refer to *any* type of sugar, whether the white stuff, high-fructose corn syrup, honey, maple syrup, or even fruit! And some even like to point out that *all* digestible carbohydrates eventually turn into sugars in the body, meaning that potatoes, rice, and squash too should be handled with great caution lest the evil leak into us.

But is sugar really as evil as some would make it out to be? Does sugar significantly increase the risk of developing cardiovascular disease or diabetes? And, while we're at it, does sugar make people fat?

The results of all studies on the possible effects of sugar in regard to cardiovascular disease are mixed, though they generally don't differentiate between different types of (added) sugar. In the 1960s and 1970s, Dr. John Yudkin published several correspondences in journals suggesting that dietary sugar may be the cause of cardiovascular disease, and he eventually went on to write a book titled *Pure, White, and Deadly* (which has recently been updated with Robert Lustig for an anti-sugar tour de force). However, in the 1969 *British Medical Journal*, Howell and Wilson published a study[39] in which they compared the diets of men with and without coronary heart disease and found no evidence to suggest a connection between dietary sugar and heart disease. In

---

[39] Howell, R.W., Wilson, D.G., "Dietary Sugar and Ischaemic Heart Disease," *British Medical Journal* (July 1969): 145-148.

1994, a study *conducted at the University of Dundee in Scotland*[40] (one of the top ranked universities in the world) concluded that "these new data for different sugar types agree with the consensus view that total sugar intake is not a major marker of coronary heart disease." (Unfortunately, this study was funded not only by the Scottish government, but also by the Sugar Bureau, but given the credentials of those involved, the findings are important.) Yet, in 2014, a sizable epidemiological study published in the *Journal of the American Medical Association Internal Medicine*[41] showed a strong positive correlation between added dietary sugar intake and cardiovascular disease. Unfortunately, we don't know *what type* of sugar correlated, but given that high-fructose corn syrup accounts for a substantial percentage of sugar intake among modern humans, it is difficult to rule out the possibility that (as has been shown in various studies) the free fructose in the corn syrup or some unknown factor (such as mercury found in high-fructose corn syrup[42]) attributable to the industrial processes used to manufacture high-fructose corn syrup could be what actually correlates with cardiovascular disease.

So the connection between sugar and cardiovascular disease is completely unproven at this point. There are a number of epidemiological studies that show conflicting results, but no well-designed human trials have been done to study the effects. It certainly is *possible* that increases in dietary sugar may be the cause of increases in cardiovascular disease. However, when we look at historical sugar consumption rates and map that to the rise in cardiovascular disease, it's not a clear match. For example, according to researcher Stephan Guyenet, the USDA reported

[40] Bolton-Smith, C., Woodward, M., "Coronary heart disease: prevalence and dietary sugars in Scotland," *Journal of Epidemiology and Community Health* (1994): 119-122.

[41] Yang et al., "Added sugar intake and cardiovascular diseases mortality among US adults," *Journal of the American Medical Association Internal Medicine* (April 2014): 516-524.

[42] Dufault et al., "Mercury from chlor-alkali plants: measured concentrations in food product sugar," *Environmental Health* (2009): 2.

that sweetener sales in the U.S. from 1822 onward show a steady and rapid rise until around 1920,[43] after which the trend has been a slower rise. The data is only for sales and doesn't indicate anything about sugar consumption that wouldn't have been recorded, such as locally produced maple syrup or honey. But if we compare that with the data from the National Institutes of Health regarding cardiovascular deaths in the United States since 1900, we don't get a good match. According to that data, cardiovascular deaths began to rise dramatically in 1900 but peaked in 1970, despite the fact that U.S. sugar consumption was *lower* in 1970 than it was in 1920.

We can also look at rates of sugar consumption by country and compare that with rates of cardiovascular disease per country to see if high sugar consumption correlates with rates of cardiovascular disease. I looked at rates of death from coronary heart disease (which is the leading form of cardiovascular disease) by country from the WHO data and compared that with per capita sugar consumption as reported by the Food and Agricultural Organization (FAO) of the U.N.[44] to see if there is any obvious correlation and I didn't find one. For example, the country with the highest mortality rates (Turkmenistan) has a per capita sugar consumption of less than 10 kg per year (for a reference point, U.S. per capita sugar consumption is 60 kg). Other countries with high cardiovascular mortality rates but low per capita sugar consumption (relatively speaking) include India, Pakistan, and Afghanistan. On the other end, there are plenty of countries with extremely low mortality rates (and not *just* because of wealth) in which per capita sugar consumption is similar or even much higher (sometimes double) the sugar consumption in the high-risk countries. Examples include Columbia, Brazil,

---

[43] http://wholehealthsource.blogspot.com/2012/02/by-2606-us-diet-will-be-100-percent.html

[44] http://faostat.fao.org

China, Panama, Peru, and France. Figure 2 shows the lack of a pattern[45].

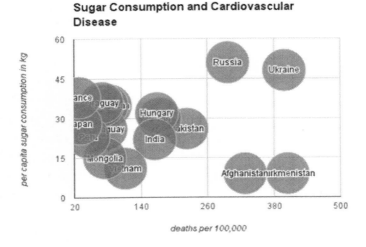

Sugar Consumption and Cardiovascular Disease

Figure 2

Could it be that sugar is a cause of cardiovascular disease? It could be. But as of yet, there is no strong evidence to support that claim. So sugar hasn't been totally exonerated, but neither has it been convicted. And since people were eating sugar of various sorts before the rise in cardiovascular disease, it seems that even *if* sugar plays a role in the development of cardiovascular disease, it is likely dependent upon other factors.

But what about sugar and diabetes? Surely, there must be a strong causative connection there.

It turns out that despite what most people *think* they know, the connection between dietary sugar and diabetes isn't proven either. Because diabetics may need to manage their sugar intake

---

[45] The data that I use here may have the same weakness as the data Keys used to argue that saturated fat may cause heart disease—namely, that it doesn't necessarily indicate precisely what people really eat. However, the utter lack of any detectable pattern in this case certainly doesn't lend credibility to the theory that sugar causes cardiovascular disease.

to avoid high blood sugar, many people mistakenly believe that dietary sugar *causes* diabetes. But the evidence actually suggests that *most* dietary sugar is not even correlated to insulin resistance or diabetes.

In 1990, a study conducted by the Dutch National Institute of Public Health and Environmental Protection[46] concluded that no link appeared between dietary sugar intake and impaired glucose tolerance. And in a randomized controlled trial conducted at the Royal Victoria Hospital in Belfast, Ireland[47] the conclusion was that "a high-sucrose intake as part of a eucaloric, weight-maintaining diet had no detrimental effect on insulin sensitivity, glycemic profiles, or measures of vascular compliance in healthy nondiabetic subjects." (Unfortunately, this study was also funded, in part, by a grant from The Sugar Bureau, but there is no reason to suspect the conclusions are anything but above board.)

On the other hand, some studies have shown a possible link between free fructose consumption and impaired insulin sensitivity. In a study published in 1980,[48] the authors concluded that humans eating very large amounts (1000 calories per day in addition to normal diet) of free fructose significantly reduced insulin sensitivity whereas the same amount of glucose did not have the same effect. But to put that into perspective, it would be impossible for anyone to eat that much fructose from real food. In fact, it would be very difficult to achieve that even if eating large amounts of high fructose corn syrup, which contains free (unbound) fructose (as opposed to bound fructose as is found in sucrose). Another human trial with more moderate

---

[46] Feskens, E.J., Kromhout, D., "Habitual dietary intake and glucose tolerance in euglycaemic men: the Zutphen Study," *International Journal of Epidemiology* (December 1990): 953-959.

[47] Black et al., "Effect of eucaloric high- and low-sucrose diets with identical macronutrient profile on insulin resistance and vascular risk: a randomized controlled trial," *Diabetes* (December 2006): 3566-3572.

[48] Beck-Nielsen et al., "Impaired cellular insulin binding and insulin sensitivity induced by high-fructose feeding in normal subjects," *American Journal of Clinical Nutrition* (February 1980): 272-278.

fructose supplementation[49] found similar, though less dramatic results. And a six-month trial published in 2012[50] found that participants who drank a liter of soda a day showed fat distribution that was indicative of potential health problems. The study claimed that the participants were drinking *sucrose*-sweetened sodas, but it is likely that 'sucrose' in this case (as often happens in these studies) really means high fructose corn syrup.

Thus far, what we can see is that there is little evidence that most sugar consumption (apart from, *maybe*, soda) leads to insulin resistance in most people. And even if someone develops insulin resistance, that doesn't mean that such a person will develop type 2 diabetes. In fact, although insulin resistance may be a risk factor, we don't know that it *causes* diabetes, and it certainly doesn't cause diabetes in all people since some people can have insulin resistance for a lifetime without ever developing diabetes. And curiously, a number of studies have demonstrated that, counterintuitively, dietary sugar may not even play a major role in glucose control in some diabetics![51]

While I was at it, I decided to run the numbers to see if there is any obvious trend between per capita sugar consumption and the prevalence of diabetes in a country. I used the FAO numbers for sugar consumption, and I got the numbers for diabetes prevalence from the IDF Diabetes Atlas.[52] What I found was no discernable trend, as seen in figure 3.

---

[49] Le et al., "A 4-wk high-fructose diet alters lipid metabolism without affecting insulin sensitivity or ectopic lipids in healthy humans," *American Journal of Clinical Nutrition* (December 2006): 1374-1379.

[50] Maersk et al., "Sucrose-sweetened beverages increase fat storage in the liver, muscle, and visceral fat depot: a 6-mo randomized intervention study," *American Journal of Clinical Nutrition* (February 2012): 283-289.

[51] Howard, B.V. and Wylie-Rossett, J., "Sugar and Cardiovascular Disease," *Circulation* (2002): 523-527.

[52] International Diabetes Federation. IDF Diabetes Atlas, 6th edn. Brussels, Belgium: International Diabetes Federation, 2013. http://www.idf.org/diabetesatlas.

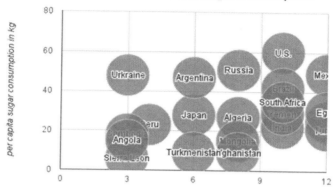

Diabetes Prevalence and Sugar Consumption

per capita sugar consumption in kg

percent of population with diabetes

Finally, is there any link between sugar intake and fatness? As far as I can tell, there does not seem to be. In 1995, the authors of an epidemiological study published in *The American Journal of Clinical Nutrition*[53] concluded that there is "no reason to associate high-sugar diets with obesity." (Unfortunately, one of the authors of the study, James O. Hill, happens to sit on the board of General Mills, Nestle, McDonald's, and a few other corporations, making his conclusions sadly fall under suspicion and once again pointing to the sad state of conflict of interest that colors most everything in the "scientific" world. However, the other author of the study, Andrew Prentice, seems to be an honorable fellow with no conflicts of interest.) In 1999, a paper in the *European Journal of Clinical Nutrition*[54] actually found that higher sugar intake correlated to leanness, stating, "Evidence showed that higher intakes of sugar were related to leanness, not obesity, and had no detrimental effects on micronutrient intakes in most people." (Though, once again, unfortunately, the lead author was affiliated

---

[53] Hill, J.O. and Prentice, A.M., "Sugar and body weight regulation," *American Journal of Clinical Nutrition* (July 1995): 2645-2735.

[54] Ruxton et al., "Guidelines for sugar consumption in Europe: is a quantitative approach justified?," *European Journal of Clinical Nutrition* (July 1999): 503-513.

with The Sugar Bureau.) And in a 2012 paper[55] that appears to be free of conflicts of interest, the authors concluded that dietary sugar intake in and of itself was not a good predictor of fatness.

Some researchers speculate that some forms of sugar—particularly free fructose—may suppress the body's natural satiety-signaling system, leading to eating beyond the actual needs of the body. The theory is that "excessive" fructose may lead to leptin resistance,[56] which means that the body won't receive satiety signals. While this is certainly a possibility that may be proved out, the body of evidence seems to suggest that naturally occurring sugars (including sucrose in refined sugar) don't have some magical capacity to produce cardiovascular disease, diabetes, or body fatness. Whether or not sugar consumption beyond caloric needs plays a role or whether possible contaminants in industrially processed sweeteners may lead to these conditions is something that may still prove out, but as of now, we don't know. Of course, the easy and conservative approach would be to avoid industrially produced sweeteners and food products.

---

[55] Song et al., "Is obesity development associated with dietary sugar intake in the U.S.?," *Nutrition* (November-December 2012): 1137-1141.

[56] Shapiro et al., "Prevention and reversal of diet-induced leptin resistance with a sugar-free diet despite high fat content," *British Journal of Nutrition* (August 2011): 390-397.

Eat Less

Of course, thus far we've only examined some of the major macronutrient shuffling recommendations made by the proponents of the diet-heart and diet-diabetes theorists. But we haven't yet looked at the dictum to eat less and move more. Because we have all been inculcated with the same messages (fatness is due to overeating and lack of movement, sickness is due to fatness, etc.), it is rare that we question the recommendations. The calories in, calories out model of weight management is practically sacrosanct; all fat people need to do is eat less and move more and their weight will drop and their health (which is assumed to be poor because of their size) will improve. It sounds so logical and simple that we believe it unquestioningly. But is it true?

To begin with, we'll explore calorie restriction. Does calorie restriction reduce cardiovascular disease and type 2 diabetes in humans? You'd sure think so, given the amount of hype. But, as it turns out, *we simply don't know*. That's because to date there haven't been any well-designed, long-term human trials to test whether calorie restriction actually reduces the incidences of cardiovascular disease or diabetes.

Of course, you'll recall from the earlier discussions that there is some evidence that sustained weight loss does sometimes correlate positively to reduced risk of these diseases. But you'll also recall that we don't know why that correlation exists. There isn't much evidence to suggest that weight loss *causes* a reduction in risk. Instead, it could be that the capacity to sustain weight loss merely indicates that a person is already at lower risk for other reasons. Or, it could be that something about the manner in which people lose weight reduces risk. In the next two sections, we're going to consider whether the standard weight loss advice (eat less, move more) are likely candidates for reducing risk.

As I have already stated, to date there are no good human trials to tell us whether calorie restriction really can offer any reduced risk of disease. Instead, we have to rely upon biomarker measurements taken from human trials as well as the outcomes from non-human primate studies to give us some indication of the likelihood of beneficial outcomes from calorie restriction.

One example of a study that is often cited as evidence that calorie restriction reduces risk is the Biosphere 2 experiment.[57] Biosphere 2 is a research facility that was sealed shut for a two-year period with eight human volunteers. The facility is intended to provide a "self-sustaining ecological system" in which all food is produced inside the facility. Due to a shortfall of food production, the human participants underwent moderate calorie restriction for the duration of the experiment, eating about 2000 calories per day each. When they were tested at intervals, they showed decreases (from baseline) in blood pressure, glucose, and insulin. Of course, this study, though interesting, is riddled with problems. Forget for a moment that it was neither blind nor random and that the sample size was very small. It is also confounded by the fact that the participants underwent *massive* lifestyle changes completely apart from moderate calorie restriction, including changes in diet composition and regular exercise in the form of daily labor.

There have been a few trials that are better designed than the Biosphere 2 experiment. Most of them are similar to a study

---

[57] Walford et al., "Alternate-day fasting and chronic disease prevention: a review of human and animal trials," *Toxicological Sciences* (1999): Supplement 61-65.

published in the *Journal of the American Medical Association* in 2006[58] in that that they compare the effects of calorie restriction (usually 25 percent below energy expenditure) versus calorie restriction and exercise (usually 12.5 percent reduction in calories and exercise designed to increase expenditure by 12.5 percent). Each typically reports the same: markers generally thought to be associated with cardiovascular health "improve," and the researchers typically conclude that calorie restriction is a good way to reduce the risk of cardiovascular disease and diabetes.

Unfortunately, what often goes unmentioned when anyone comments on these studies is the *glaring* evidence that long-term calorie restriction has some undesirable side effects. In nearly every study, including the Biosphere 2 report and multiple six-month trials, the published data shows a significant reduction in basal body temperature, pulse, energy expenditure, and T3 (the "active" thyroid hormone)—all of which indicate lowered metabolic rate. The researchers typically seem to think that these reductions may explain the supposed, though entirely unproven, lifespan-increasing effects of calorie restriction. But what they are missing is the obvious; lowered metabolic rate is a well-known adaptive strategy that the body utilizes during times of starvation. Lowered basal metabolic rate is well documented among those suffering from restrictive eating disorders,[59] and the landmark Minnesota Starvation Experiment demonstrated that a state of semi-starvation produced by feeding men 1600 calories a day produced lowered basal metabolic rate in addition to a long list of very unpleasant symptoms. The Minnesota Starvation Experiment was so successful in demonstrating the *negative*

[58] Heilbronn et al., "Effect of 6-month calorie restriction on biomarkers of longevity, metabolic adaptation and oxidative stress in overweight subjects," *Journal of the American Medical Association* (2006): 1539-1548.

[59] One such example of a study demonstrating the link is Polito et al., "Basal metabolic rate in anorexia nervosa: relation to body composition and leptin concentrations," *The American Journal of Clinical Nutrition* (June 2000): 1495-1502.

effects of calorie restriction that to repeat the experiment now would be considered unethical.

While low T3 levels are not an indicator of clinical hypothyroidism, it does indicate something amiss, and it is therefore given the name euthyroid sick syndrome (ESS). According to the Merck Manual, ESS is often seen as the result of various conditions, including fasting, starvation, protein deficiency, and anorexia nervosa. And, importantly, ESS is associated with *increased risk* for cardiovascular disease.[60] In other words, chronic calorie restriction may not be the best way to reduce the risk of cardiovascular disease.

What about diabetes? Does low T3 potentially have some connection with diabetes as well? Although not as clear as with cardiovascular disease, it would seem that there may be some association here as well. According to an article published in *Clinical Diabetes* in 2000,[61] thyroid disorders, including ESS, are *much* more common among diabetics than in the general population. Of course, low T3 could be the *result* of diabetes rather than a contributing factor, but until there is more research into the matter, I'd say that it's a little too early to make a strong case for any practice that lowers T3 as a way to *lower* the risk of a condition in which low T3 is common.

The truth is that although calorie restriction has gotten a lot of positive press in recent years, there are *no* human trials that *actually* demonstrate a benefit while at the same time there is quite a lot of evidence (including the Minnesota Starvation Experiment, lots of research into anorexia nervosa, and even the research that purports to demonstrate that calorie restriction in humans has benefits) that chronic calorie restriction has negative impacts on health in humans.

The idea that calorie restriction has benefits got started when it was noticed that restricting calories seemed to increase the

---

[60] Iervasi et al., "Low-T3 Syndrome; A Strong Prognostic Predictor of Death in Patients With Heart Disease," *Circulation* (January 2003): 708-713.

[61] Wu, P., "Thyroid Disease and Diabetes," *Clinical Diabetes* (Winter 2000).

lifespan of *yeast*.[62] Subsequently, tests were done on other species with mixed results. For example, studies showed that calorie restriction increased life expectancy in some species of specially bred mice but not in wild mice.

In 2009, the researchers of a long-term study on calorie restriction in rhesus monkeys published a paper in *Science*[63] in which it was claimed that calorie restriction prevented early onset of disease. However, as blogger Sandy Szwarc has pointed out, the report was deeply flawed. For one thing, the "calorie restricted" monkeys were not, in fact, calorie restricted in the normal sense in which the term is used. They received 30 percent fewer calories than the control group, but the control group received 20 percent more calories than the "usual" diet. Do the math and we find out that the "calorie restricted" monkeys were eating 84 percent of "usual" calories, which is quite different than 70 percent, which is what we might think at a casual reading of the report.

But the relatively modest restriction and the fairly substantial *overfeeding* of the control group is not the major flaw. The report claims that the restricted monkeys had a much lower rate of death—*but only after excluding a large number of monkeys from the restricted group who died*. In other words, they cooked the books. They manipulated the numbers by suggesting that the restricted monkeys who died of things other than heart attacks and other "allowable" diseases shouldn't count. So they excluded the calorie-restricted monkeys who died from things like gastritis, injuries, and endometriosis. When deaths from all causes are included, there was *no statistically significant difference* between the two groups. Another way to interpret the data is that calorie restriction is correlated with higher risk of death from other causes. And for all we know, had the monkeys who died from

---

[62] Lin et al., "Calorie restriction extends yeast life span by lowering the level of NADH," *Genes and Development* (January 2004): 12-16.

[63] Weindruch et al., "Caloric Restriction Delays Disease Onset and Mortality in Rhesus Monkeys," *Science* (July 2009): 201-204.

other causes lived, they too would have died of all the same things as the well-fed monkeys.

Calorie restriction may extend the lifespan of yeast and some lab mice, but when it comes to primates, the benefits are not so clear. In fact, it would appear that in rhesus monkeys, calorie restriction may contribute to greater risk of death from some causes. And in humans, it would seem that the main measurable effect of calorie restriction is lowered basal metabolic rate and low serum T3, both of which are commonly seen in starvation.

Then the question becomes, how many calories are needed to avoid starvation (or semi-starvation, if you prefer)? How many calories are necessary to maintain a healthy basal metabolic rate and serum T3 levels? The answer seems to be that it depends.

In the Minnesota Starvation Experiment, the researchers found that prior to initiating the starvation phase, the participants required 3200 calories a day to maintain weight and function. Then, for six months, the men were restricted to an average of 1600 calories a day, which produced a 40 percent reduction in basal metabolic rate. Afterward, the men had to eat a minimum of 4000 calories a day for nine months, gaining back lost weight *plus* 10 percent in order to restore metabolic health and eventually restore original weight (i.e., the additional 10 percent weight came off as a result of continuing to "overeat," *not* as a result of dieting).

On the other hand, we have examples of cultures in which heart disease and diabetes are (or were at the time of study) unheard of, and in some of those cultures the men are able to seemingly sustain themselves on less than 3200 calories a day. For example, the Kitavans were studied in the 1980s because they were found to have virtually no "modern diseases" and because they still ate their traditional diet. It was found that they ate a diet very high in carbohydrates and almost all of the dietary fat was saturated. The average daily caloric intake among adults was 2200. The daily calories weren't broken down by sex, but we can assume that the men were eating more than 2200 calories a day while the women were eating less. (Interestingly, though smoking is generally considered to be a major risk factor for disease, the Kitavans were found to be smoking heavily.)

The Tokelauans are another example of a modern people who were studied while they were still eating their traditional diet and who were virtually free of "modern diseases." The Tokelauans were found to eat 54 percent of their calories from fat, almost all of it saturated. The men ate 2520 calories a day and the women ate 2100 calories a day.

Although this information isn't a comprehensive study on the matter, it does demonstrate that none of these people were consistently eating 1600 (or fewer) calories a day as many calorie restriction advocates suggest. The Americans studied in the Minnesota Starvation Experiment seemed to need considerably more calories than the traditional islanders (the Kitavans and Tokelauans), which would seem to suggest that perhaps there is some hitherto unknown factor that contributed to the increased caloric requirement of the Americans.

And finally, although, as we've already established, weight is not a good indicator of health (or lack thereof), it is worth considering whether calorie restriction is even a useful means for shedding fat since it is often promoted as such. Of course, we are all familiar with the so-called yo-yo syndrome in which dieters gain back lost weight *and then some* over several years. Why that might be so is elucidated by the revelation from the calorie restriction studies that calorie restriction produces a reduction in basal metabolic rate. In other words, the body slows down to save its life in times of starvation.

The calories in, calories out model of weight management has been around since at least the early 1900s when a German doctor theorized that the number of dietary calories consumed, regardless of the source or type, could predict the weight gain or loss. The theory is so simple and so easy to market that many people believe that it is absolutely true.

And, to some extent, it *is* true. In science it is generally believed that energy cannot be created or destroyed; it can only be transformed. So in some manner or another it would seem that weight gain or loss can be predicted by the number of calories taken in versus the number of calories used. But properly calculating the number of calories used turns out to be a tricky business. Why? Well, for one thing, the human metabolism adjusts in accordance with how much is eaten and what type of foods are eaten, among other things.

The calorie restriction interpretation of calories in, calories out hasn't fared well when tested over the years. In recent years, several studies have tested whether or not all calories are really equal, and it turns out, they don't seem to be. In 2003, a pilot study at Harvard[64] examined three groups: low-fat diet, low-carbohydrate diet, and low-carbohydrate diet with extra calories. What they found was that the latter two groups both lost *more* weight than the low-fat group, despite the fact that the third group was eating 300 calories more a day than the low-fat group. However, unfortunately, the low-carbohydrate groups showed the most inflammation, and inflammation is often an indicator of disease conditions. So low-carbohydrate may not necessarily be the panacea that it is often made out to be.

Yet even the *type* of calories consumed may be less significant than other factors, including those that have led to what is known as the setpoint theory, which states that each body has a setpoint from which one can lose or gain a small amount of weight with relative ease, but beyond that the body will strive to maintain weight by making adjustments (that aren't fully understood). The theory states that the setpoint for an individual may be subject to various factors, which may include drugs and environmental factors and perhaps even the *types* of foods eaten. It is possible that the setpoint may even be subject to change due to periods of starvation or semi-starvation.

In support of the setpoint theory, we have a few important experiments. First, there was the Minnesota Starvation Experiment in which participants were placed on a six-month

---

[64] Greene, P., Willett, W., et al. "Pilot 12-week feeding weight loss comparison: low-fat vs. low-carbohydrate (ketogenic) diets," *Obesity Research* (2003):A23.

semi-starvation diet of an average of 1600 calories a day. The goal was to cause the men to lose 25 percent of their starting weight. However, despite severe measures, including some men being restricted to as little as 1000 calories a day at times in an effort to eke out further weight loss, the men didn't reach their targets. They came close, but in the last month of the semi-starvation phase of the experiment, the men stopped losing weight. In fact, some even *gained* weight despite being on severe restrictions. Not surprisingly, the average metabolic rate of the men dropped by 40 percent during the semi-starvation phase.

Once the men began eating again, averaging at least 4000 calories a day for many months (and sometimes more than 10,000 calories a day), they eventually gained back their lost weight *plus* 10 percent. Importantly, however, they eventually restored their initial weight *when they continued to eat large quantities of food for long periods of time.*

In contrast with the Minnesota Starvation Experiment, we have the Vermont Prison studies. In the 1960s, Dr. Ethan Sims of the University of Vermont began an overfeeding experiment with university students. For months on end, the students ate many times (2-3 times) their normal amount of food, but they were unable to gain more than 12 percent of their starting weight. Dr. Sims gave up on the experiment in a university environment, convinced that an increase in "spontaneous movements" on the part of the free-roaming students was to blame for the stalled weight gain.

Sims next began a series of experiments in the Vermont state prison.[65] He enlisted lean volunteers to partake in an overfeeding study. Initially he kept track of the number of calories required for the men to maintain their normal weights, which was between 3000 and 4000 calories a day. That was followed by a period of intense overeating in which the men were to reduce their activity

---

[65] Sims et al., "Experimental obesity in man: a progress report," *Israel Journal of Medical Science* (June 1972): 813-814.

and eat anywhere between 6000 and 10,000 calories a day with the intention of gaining 25 percent of their starting weight.

Many of the men simply could not reach their goal no matter how hard they tried. And, in a mirror image of the starvation experiments, Sims found that during the overfeeding phase, the men's metabolic rates increased by 50 percent. What is more, in order for the men to maintain the increased weight, they had to continue to eat extremely large amounts of food—much more than had previously been necessary to maintain their starting weight, which isn't surprising given the dramatic increase in metabolic rate.

In the 1990s, a man named Rudolph Leibel, the man who discovered the hormone leptin, performed experiments at Rockefeller University[66] to study the setpoint theory in humans. He and his colleagues found that the participants studied in a tightly controlled environment maintained their weights within a narrow range even when overfed. In fact, once substantial weight was gained, the participants' metabolisms began to increase *significantly*. Outside of *extreme* circumstances (such as the Minnesota Starvation Experiment or the Vermont prison studies), most people don't gain or lose much weight just by eating more or less—at least according to Leibel's research.

Of course, many dieters can and do lose weight by subjecting themselves to semi-starvation conditions (keep in mind that many modern diets can make the Minnesota Starvation Experiment 1600 calories a day look downright gluttonous!), but it is rare for calorie restriction to result in sustained weight loss unless the calorie restriction is also maintained, which may come with its own set of symptoms in time. In the typical modern context, dieters may restrict for a few months in order to lose weight, followed by a resumption of normal calories (or perhaps sub-normal, but still more than the initial restriction). Because dieters rarely eat enough to restore their pre-diet metabolic rate, the result is that with a suppressed metabolic rate even "normal"

---

[66] Gibbs, W.W., Interview with Rudolph L. Leibel, *Scientific American* (August 1996).

amounts of food will continue to lead to slow weight gain. It is reasonable to suggest that cyclical patterns of calorie restriction followed by "normal" eating will result in ever-slowing metabolisms, meaning "normal" eating will continue to pack on more pounds. In a paper written from the University of California at Los Angeles,[67] the authors conclude, "there is little support for the notion that diets lead to lasting weight loss or health benefits."

In summary, despite the exaggerated claims as to the benefits of calorie restriction, for the majority of people, sustained calorie restriction is not possible nor does it yield actual benefits. Sustained calorie restriction produces a state of starvation that eventually produces death or abandonment of the practice. Once calorie restriction is abandoned, the lowered metabolic rate will result in weight gain, often well beyond pre-diet weight, and a "worsening" of the biomarkers associated with various disease states. And, as we've now seen, even when biomarkers are "improved" in the starved state, at least one (low T3) is actually associated with disease states.

Might some people benefit from (very) modest reductions in caloric intake? Sure, that seems plausible, particularly if a large number of restricted calories are from industrially produced free fructose, which has at least some evidence to back the idea that it could contribute to disease states. So perhaps a reduction in soda consumption *may* be helpful for some people. But restricting calories and producing states of semi-starvation have largely been demonstrated to be counterproductive to health.

---

[67] Mann et al., "Medicare's search for effective obesity treatments: diets are not the answer.," *American Psychologist* (April 2007): 220-233.

Move More

What about the dictum to move more? Surely, exercise is always a good thing. After all, just about *everyone* seems to agree about that. Yet the actual story seems to be more nuanced. Let's take a look.

To begin with, is there any evidence that movement and exercise are closely associated with reduced risk of cardiovascular disease and type 2 diabetes? Yes, there is. There is quite a lot of it, in fact. Numerous studies demonstrate a clear link between physical activity and fewer incidences of disease.

What is important to note, however, is that different types of physical activity may offer different benefits, and more is not always better. In study after study, the evidence is clear: those who move fare better than those who don't. Generally, those who are highly sedentary are at the highest risk. Of course, we don't know if being sedentary is a *cause* of disease or if it is a symptom. But given the body of evidence, it seems likely that physical activity has good potential to be beneficial.

Steady-state cardio exercise (jogging, cycling, swimming, elliptical machines, etc.) for more than 30 minutes has been shown to produce an increase in stress hormones and a decrease in serum T3.[68] And, significantly, one study[69] showed that in prolonged exercise, the "changes in peripheral thyroid hormone metabolism [decrease in T3 and increase in reverse T3] are similar to those found in starvation." Steady state cardio exercise for 30 minutes or more produces a catabolic state,[70] meaning that muscle begins to break down. Since lean muscle mass has benefits for health, including insulin sensitivity and cardiovascular health, prolonged catabolism is counterproductive for health.

However, other forms of movement, including both low-intensity exercise[71] (walking, standing, etc.) and short-term high intensity interval training[72] have been shown to offer benefits for insulin sensitivity and serum T3 levels.

What is notable about the mentions of exercise in the literature pertaining to risk reduction is that the benefits are had completely

---

[68] Neto et al., "Decreased serum T3 after an exercise session is independent of glucocorticoid peak," *Hormone and Metabolic Research* (November 2013): 893-899.

[69] O'Connell et al., "Changes in serum concentrations of 3,3',5'-triiodothyronine and 3,5,3'-triiodothyronine during prolonged moderate exercise," *Journal of Clinical Endocrinology and Metabolism* (August 1979): 242-246.

[70] Dohm et al., "Protein metabolism during endurance exercise," *Federation Proceedings* (February 1985): 348-352; Lindholm et al., "Hormone anabolic/catabolic balance in female endurance athletes," *Gynecologic and Obstetric Investigation* (1993): 176-180.

[71] Kishimoto et al., "Effect of short-term low-intensity exercise on insulin sensitivity, insulin secretion, and glucose and lipid metabolism in non-obese Japanese type 2 diabetic patients," *Hormone and Metabolic Research* (January 2002): 27-31; Newsom et al., "A single session of low-intensity exercise is sufficient to enhance insulin sensitivity into the next day in obese adults," *Diabetes Care* (September 2013): 2516-2522.

[72] Babraj et al., "Extremely short duration high intensity interval training substantially improves insulin action in young healthy males," *BMC Endocrine Disorders* (January 2009): 3; Shaban et al., "The effects of a 2 week modified high intensity interval training program on the homeostatic model of insulin resistance (HOMA-IR) in adults with type 2 diabetes," *Journal of Sports Medicine and Physical Fitness* (April 2014): 203-209; Richards et al., "Short-term sprint interval training increases insulin sensitivity in healthy adults but does not affect the thermogenic response to β-adrenergic stimulation," *Journal of Physiology* (August 2010): 2961-2972.

independent of changes in BMI, weight, or fatness. In other words, it may be possible to have health benefits from modest movement without having to lose weight. And the amount of time necessary to achieve these benefits is also modest. In fact, on the low end, in one of the studies, insulin sensitivity improved significantly with only 16 minutes of high-intensity interval training *per two weeks*. On the other hand, with moderate-intensity movement, benefits in cardiovascular health and risk reduction for diabetes can be seen in 30 minutes of movement several times a week.[73]

As we've already seen, movement that may offer health benefits needn't produce change in weight. Unfortunately, since weight is often used as a measure of health both by the individual and by health care professionals, a common approach to physical activity is to do it as a means to lose weight. Yet it turns out that such an approach can be counterproductive when poorly executed.

You'll recall that I noted earlier that some forms of exercise (steady-state cardio for more than 30 minutes at a time) can produce unwanted metabolic effects such as reductions in serum T3 levels that mimic starvation. Increases in lean muscle mass, which may come about through some forms of exercise coupled with adequate nutrition and rest, may result in a slight elevation in basal metabolic rate, which may help to support sustained leanness. However, when exercise is taken to an extreme (as in long bouts of steady-state cardio), the basal metabolic rate may become suppressed.[74]

So in conclusion, it would seem that *some* exercise, particularly low-intensity exercise and very short bursts of high-intensity exercise (with adequate rest days), can potentially improve health.

---

[73] Thompson et al., "Exercise and Physical Activity in the Prevention and Treatment of Atherosclerotic Cardiovascular Disease," *Circulation* (2003): 3109-3116.

[74] Speakman, J.R. and Selman, C., "Physical activity and resting metabolic rate," *Proceedings of the Nutritional Society* (August 2003): 621-634.

However, too much exercise or the wrong types of exercise may actually be counterproductive. The most important takeaway, perhaps, is that the forms of exercise that can yield health benefits are the types of exercise that do not necessarily have any significant impact on BMI or body composition. The evidence is mounting that the use of BMI or even fatness is not a valid measure of health.

What's Causing Illness

We've been told that there is a worldwide "obesity epidemic." In other words, we are told that people are dying of fatness. But as we've started to see, that's not really true. Instead, people are dying from cardiovascular disease, complications from type 2 diabetes, cancer, and other conditions. Although many have attempted to pin the blame on fatness and have succeeded in convincing the public of that supposed fact, the reality remains that there is no evidence that fatness is to blame for these conditions.

Furthermore, as we've seen, the standard dictum of "eat less and move more" falls short, especially when the usual advice is followed to an extreme (and, hopefully, we've also started to see that what is generally considered to be moderate is really more toward the extreme end of things). Not only does this advice fall short, but it may be counterproductive since calorie restriction and overexercise can lead to low serum T3, high cortisol, and other indicators of stress, inflammation, and poor health as are seen during starvation.

The truth is that despite the fact that various organizations (including the CDC, the WHO, the American Heart Association, and the American Diabetes Association, among others) proclaim that it is possible to reduce risk through *individual* dietary and exercise changes, the evidence seems to suggest that, at the very least, there's a lot more to the story than we've been led to believe. While it appears that *some* people *may* be able to reduce risk through dietary changes and moderate increases in physical activity, those recommendations simply aren't sufficient to actually reduce rates of cardiovascular disease and diabetes like they are *supposed* to, according to the experts.

As we've already seen, rates of diabetes and cardiovascular disease continue to rise worldwide. Yet we also see that according to NHANES, Americans are following the dietary guidelines. The weight-loss companies such as NutriSystem, Weight Watchers, and Jenny Craig are raking in $60 billion per year as millions of people desperately fork over their money, hoping that they can lose weight. Bariatric surgery continues to grow (the irony) at an impressive (and frightening) pace, with 150,000 procedures performed each year in the United States, causing 150,000 people to comply with *extremely* low-calorie diets. According to the U.S. Department of Health and Human Services, rates of smoking in the U.S. have decreased dramatically, nearly halving since 1985. And a report from the Institute of Health Metrics and Evaluation [75] found that Americans are exercising considerably more over the last decade.

Something isn't adding up. If people are doing some of the "right" things that they've been told to do and yet the "problems" that the advice was said to remedy persist or continue to increase, it would seem that either the advice wasn't very good or, at the very least, the advice was *insufficient*. There may be other factors that haven't been part of the discussion up to now.

I decided to investigate the literature in order to see if I could find any known possible factors that could explain the situation. What I wanted to find was anything that is known or suspected to contribute to cardiovascular disease or diabetes. Furthermore, given that we are all, seemingly, getting fatter, I wanted to know if there are any factors that could both explain increases in disease *and* increases in waistlines. I figured that if anything could explain

---

[75] Institute for Health Metrics and Evaluation. The State of US Health: Innovations, Insights, and Recommendations from the Global Burden of Disease Study. Seattle, WA: IHME, 2013.

both increases in diseases and increasing weight, then *that* would be something worth investigating in more detail.

Interestingly, it wasn't hard to find factors that can both contribute to increases in disease and growing weight. Among the factors are psychological stress, insufficient sleep, radiation exposure, pharmaceutical drugs, and environmental chemical exposure, all of which we'll explore in more detail in the sections that follow.

Before we continue, I want to reiterate something from earlier in the book. One of the biggest risk factors for cardiovascular disease and diabetes is increasing age, and the worldwide population is growing increasingly older. This simple fact alone might account for much of the increases in disease, and so it is important that we don't overstate the "problem." Furthermore, to be clear, I am *not* proposing that diet and physical activity don't contribute to the development of cardiovascular disease and diabetes. Rather, I am merely observing that the magnitude of their contributions seems to have been grossly overstated and is likely very misunderstood, and I am stating that there may be *other* contributing factors that are not receiving enough attention. Whether or not the factors that we will explore in the following sections are the most important or the *only* factors worth considering is not something I know. I am merely reporting what I have found for your consideration and to hopefully increase the scope of the public discussion on the matter.

Psychological Stress

When we speak of stress, most of us conjure the image or feeling of too many responsibilities, crying babies, phones ringing, stacks of unpaid bills, visiting in-laws, and so forth. In the popular use of the term, "stress" is a highly subjective, vague term. But in scientific terms, it is possible to measure stress through the effects on the body.

There are two types of stress: acute and chronic. As long as acute stress episodes are relatively infrequent, there is evidence that at least some acute stress may be beneficial. For example, both high-intensity interval training and weight lifting produce stress in the body, but studies show that as long as adequate nutrition and rest are included in the equation, these types of exercise can offer health benefits. And there is the old adage that says that "what doesn't kill you makes you stronger," which states what many of us have experienced: infrequent episodes of acute stress, including what we might term "psychological stress," can lead to perceived benefits over time.

Chronic stress, however, is the major type of stress that is connected with health declines. Studies, including one published in 2013,[76] demonstrate that psychological stress predicts lowered immunity. The ways in which stress can lower immunity include changes in "glucocorticoids, catecholamines, endogenous

---

[76] Jaremka et al., "Marital distress prospectively predicts poorer cellular immune function," *Psychoneuroendocrinology* (November 2013): 2713-2719.

opioids, and pituitary hormones."[77] Of special note are the glucocorticoid cortisol and the catecholamine norepinephrine, both of which are elevated during stress and which can produce undesirable effects when they remain elevated for long periods of time. Stress weakens the blood-brain barrier, allowing chemicals and organisms into the brain that wouldn't otherwise be able to cross over. Chronic stress also reduces neuroplasticity in the brain, meaning that the innate adaptability of the body becomes impaired. And the high levels of cortisol seen during stress inhibit the conversion of T4 to T3, the "active" thyroid hormone.

All in all, there's a lot of overlap between chronic stress of any kind and the effects of starvation or overexercise. In fact, starvation and overexercise are two forms of chronic stress. And all forms of chronic stress are, not surprisingly, linked to various disease states. In particular, in this book, we'll look at the links between stress and cardiovascular disease and diabetes.

Stress has long been documented to have a connection with cardiovascular disease. According to a paper published in *Nature Reviews, Cardiology* in 2012[78]:

Epidemiological data show that chronic stress predicts the occurrence of coronary heart disease (CHD). Employees who experience work-related stress and individuals who are socially isolated or lonely have an increased risk of a first CHD event. In addition, short-term emotional stress can act as a trigger of cardiac events among individuals with advanced atherosclerosis. A stress-specific coronary syndrome known as transient left ventricular apical ballooning cardiomyopathy, or stress (Takotsubo) cardiomyopathy, also exists. Among patients with CHD, acute psychological stress has been shown

---

[77] Dantzer, R. and Kelley, K.W., "Stress and immunity: an integrated view of relationships between the brain and the immune system," *Life Science* (1989): 1995-2008.

[78] Steptoe, A. and Kivimaki, M., "Stress and cardiovascular disease," *Nature Reviews. Cardiology* (April 2012): 360-370.

to induce transient myocardial ischemia and long-term stress can increase the risk of recurrent CHD events and mortality.

Although the precise mechanisms by which stress may contribute to cardiovascular disease are not known, the correlation is strong, which has given rise to various theories. One such theory is simply that chronic stress produces inflammation and that inflammation, over time, leads to heart disease.[79] Whatever the case, an increasing number of researchers are seeing the apparent connection between stress and cardiovascular disease.

Stress has also long been associated with type 2 diabetes. A handful of epidemiological studies and published papers [80] demonstrate a positive correlation between psychological stress and the development of type 2 diabetes. Of course, correlation does not prove causation, but it is worth noting that there is a link, and as concluded by the authors of a study published in Diabetic Medicine in 2013,[81] "[s]elf-perceived permanent stress is an important long-term predictor of diagnosed diabetes, independently of socio-economic status, BMI, and other conventional [t]ype 2 diabetes risk factors."

The specific mechanisms by which stress may contribute to disease have not been well studied. However, the correlation is well reported. And so it is at least worth considering the likely causes of stress.

Does stress increase fatness? Well, it seems that it might. There are a number of interesting studies that demonstrate a link.

---

[79] Black, P.H. and Garbutt, L.D., "Stress, inflammation and cardiovascular disease," *Journal of Psychosomatic Research* (January 2002): 1-23.

[80] A good example is the following: Pouwer et al., "Does emotional stress cause type 2 diabetes mellitus? A review from the European Depression in Diabetes (EDID) Research Consortium," *Discovery Medicine* (February 2010): 112-118.

[81] Novak et al., "Perceived stress and incidence of Type 2 diabetes: a 35-year follow-up study of middle-aged Swedish men," *Diabetic Medicine* (January 2013): 8-16.

In a review paper from the New York Obesity Research Center,[82] the authors found that chronic stress alters metabolic activity, which leads to both increased fatness and metabolic diseases. A study conducted at the University of Maryland[83] found that nurses who worked longer hours were more likely to be fatter than nurses who worked shorter hours. In an article from the Athens University Medical School in Greece,[84] the authors report that chronic stress leads to a vicious cycle in which metabolic derangement can increase fat tissue, which can further increase physiological stress. And in Sweden, researchers even found that those living near airports and exposed to aircraft noise over long periods of time are fatter,[85] particularly around the middle, which the researchers attribute to stress from the noise.

In the 2011 edition of *Monitor on Psychology*, the American Psychological Association (APA) published the results of a survey on stress in the United States.[86] The findings include that stress in the U.S. is on the rise with 44 percent of survey participants reporting increasing stress. The next year, researchers from Carnegie Mellon University published the results of their surveys[87] indicating much the same, though they quantified the increases in stress as being as much as 30 percent among some people during the last three decades.

---

[82] Bose et al., "Stress and obesity: the role of the hypothalamic-pituitary-adrenal axis in metabolic disease," *Current Opinion in Endocrinology, Diabetes, and Obesity* (October 2009): 340-346.

[83] Han et al., "Job stress and work schedules in relation to nurse obesity," *Journal of Nursing Administration* (November 2011): 488-495.

[84] Kyrou et al., "Stress, visceral obesity, and metabolic complications," *Annals of the New York Academy of Sciences* (November 2006): 77-110.

[85] Eriksson et al., "Long-Term Aircraft Noise Exposure and Body Mass Index, Waist Circumference, and Type 2 Diabetes: A Prospective Study," *Environmental Health Perspectives* (July 2014): 687-694.

[86] Clay, R.A., "Stressed in America," *Monitor on Psychology* (January 2011): 60.

[87] Cohen, S. and Janicki-Deverts, D., "Who's Stressed? Distributions of Psychological Stress in the United States in Probability Samples from 1983, 2006, and 2009," *Journal of Applied Social Psychology* (2012): 1320-1334.

What are the issues that people report as being the most stressful? Topping the list in the APA surveys are money, work, "the economy," and family responsibilities. Also included are relationships, personal health concerns, housing costs, job stability, health problems affecting family, and personal safety.

Of course, we all know that, by and large, modern humans don't tend to be very skilled when it comes to dealing with stress, but my guess is that our skill hasn't significantly decreased in the past 30 years. Instead, I'd guess that social and economic conditions contribute significantly to the increases in stress. This guess is supported by the fact that money, work, and "the economy" comprise the top three stresses reported to the APA, while housing costs and job stability are other major stressors.

It is possible, of course, for individuals to learn better skills for dealing with stress, and those skills can make a difference in individual health and well-being. A number of studies have reported that stress reduction techniques may be effective in reducing stress hormones such as cortisol, which, when elevated, can impair immunity.[88] Reductions in stress have been linked to reduced risk of cardiovascular events.[89] And stress reduction can potentially improve glycemic control in diabetics.[90]

However, given the nature of the major stressors modern humans are facing, it is also possible that a reprioritization of social values may be called for. If money, work, and "the economy" are the top three stressors, then perhaps a society that values health and well-being would want to consider ways in which to ease those burdens. But then again, there's not a lot of

[88] Cruess et al., "Cognitive-behavioral stress management reduces serum cortisol by enhancing benefit finding among women being treated for early stage breast cancer," *Psychosomatic Medicine* (May-June 2000): 304-308.

[89] Campbell et al., "An investigation of the benefits of stress management within a cardiac rehabilitation population," *Journal of Cardiopulmonary Rehabilitation and Prevention* (September-October 2012): 296-304.

[90] Surwit et al., "Stress management improves long-term glycemic control in type 2 diabetes," *Diabetes Care* (January 2002): 30-34.

money to be made in an honest attempt to rehumanize social priorities.

Sleep

Another major stressor that often goes overlooked is sleep deprivation. According to a Gallup poll conducted in late 2013, 40 percent of American adults get less than seven hours of sleep a night. Many sleep experiments demonstrate that adults require *at least* seven hours of sleep per night, and many suggest that a daytime nap may also be required to maintain health. Of particular interest is not only the *length* of sleep, but also the *rhythm* of the sleep. The normal pattern of sleep in modern times is for people to lie down in the late evening and then rise in the early morning, hopefully sleeping for a single stretch of as many hours as possible—apparently not enough. But researchers such as Thomas Wehr, science emeritus at the National Institutes of Mental Health, have found that the *natural* circadian rhythms of humans predispose them to sleep in a biphasic pattern of 4 hours early in the night and 4 hours in the early morning with a period of wakefulness in between. Roger Ekirch, a historian from Virginia Tech, has written a book, *At Day's Close*, in which he cites extensive historical research that supports the notion that this biphasic pattern of sleep has long been the normal pattern for humans and that it has been valued for offering many benefits.

Also of note is that adults are not the only ones who are sleep deprived. Children too are sleeping less and less. According to the authors of *NurtureShock*, children are getting an hour less sleep today than 30 years ago. According to a study conducted by

University of Kentucky researcher Fred Danner,[91] children aren't getting much sleep. Half of teens in the U.S. are getting less than 7 hours of sleep per night (on weeknights). It's bad enough for adults, but for children it's even worse. Although a recent review published in *Sleep*[92] points out that to date there exist no evidence-based guidelines for sleep needs, it also points out that what guidelines do exist suggest that children ages 5 to 10 need 10 to 11 hours of sleep a day, and teens need 8.5 to 9+ hours of sleep a day, which means that half of teens may be getting shortchanged by 2 hours of needed sleep per night.

What are the impacts of sleep deficits? In the same review published in *Sleep*, the authors look at the outcomes of six studies conducted by the National Sleep Foundation that each demonstrate a measurable negative impact of sleep deprivation, even when people are deprived of just a single hour of sleep in a night. Both cognitive function and behavioral response were measured and found to be negatively impacted by lack of sufficient sleep. And some researchers such as Fred Danner are recommending later school start times in order to correct for some of the problems associated with sleep deprivation. For example, half of the accidents caused by falling asleep at the wheel are caused by teens in the United States, and some researchers suggest that this can be corrected by allowing them to sleep more.

What are the physiological effects of sleep deprivation? Not surprisingly, they look a lot like other types of chronic stress. Studies show that sleep loss results in cortisol pattern dysregulation. They also show that sleep loss results in *decreased*

---

[91] Danner, F., "Adolescent sleep and daytime functioning: a national study." *Sleep*. 2000;23:A199–200.

[92] Matricciani, L., Blunden, S., Rigney, G., Williams, M.T., Olds, T.S., "Children's sleep needs: is there sufficient evidence to recommend optimal sleep for children?" *Sleep* 2013;36(4):527-534.

insulin sensitivity.[93] And while the initial effect of sleep loss is actually *increased* serum T3 levels (likely as a means to energize the body), after two nights without sleep, sleep serum T3 levels fall below normal[94] as we see in any chronic stress situation. Whether this pattern plays out in the case of chronic sleep deficit isn't known, but it seems likely. This mimics the pattern of stress noted by famed stress researcher Hans Selye that he termed the General Adaptive Syndrome in which initial stages of resistance to stress (such as elevated T3 levels) eventually give way to exhaustion (lowered T3).

Does a lack of sleep correlate with increased incidence of cardiovascular disease and diabetes? It turns out that, yes, there is a correlation. In the Nurses' Health Study, it was found that women who received eight hours of sleep a night had the fewest cases of heart disease. The less sleep women got, the greater the likelihood of cardiovascular disease. (Interestingly, likelihood of cardiovascular disease also increased with nine or more hours of sleep per night, which reinforces the importance of viewing the data as mere correlation, not suggesting causation.) And two studies[95] showed a correlation between sleep and likelihood of type 2 diabetes, where the lowest risk was found among those who slept between seven and eight hours each night.

Interestingly, researchers have started to look at the relationship between sleep (or lack thereof) and fatness—usually suggesting that lack of sleep may be a cause of fatness, which they claim is a killer. Obviously, I disagree with the notion that fatness is a killer, but it is interesting that insufficient sleep is positively

---

[93] Leproult, R, and Van Cauter, E., "Role of Sleep and Sleep Loss in Hormonal Release and Metabolism," *Endocrine Development* (2010): 11-21.

[94] Ilan et al., "Prolonged sleep-deprivation induced disturbed liver functions serum lipid levels, and hyperphosphatemia," *European Journal of Clinical Investigation* (November 1992): 740-743.

[95] Gottlieb, D.J., Punjabi, N.M., Newman, A.B., et al. "Association of sleep time with diabetes mellitus and impaired glucose tolerance," *Arch Intern Med.* 2005;165:863–7;Yaggi, H.K., Araujo, A.B., McKinlay, J.B., "Sleep duration as a risk factor for the development of type 2 diabetes." *Diabetes Care.* 2006;29:657–61.

correlated to disease states *and* increased fatness. In a meta-analysis published in *Sleep* in 2008,[96] the authors looked at data including over 600,000 people worldwide, and they concluded that in both children and adults insufficient sleep is positively correlated with increased fatness. And there has been at least one controlled, human trial[97] showing that decreased sleep can result in a loss of lean muscle mass whereas adequate sleep can result in an increase in the ratio of lean mass to fat. The implication is that sleep deprivation favors muscle catabolism over burning fat, which isn't a good thing.

Although it is impossible to determine causation, the close link between lack of sleep and a variety of diseases plus the link with increased fatness at least suggests that insufficient sleep *may* be a common contributing factor to all these conditions. That coupled with the fact that insufficient sleep is shown to significantly impair cognitive function and behavior suggests that sleep really ought to be a subject of major public discussion.

Given the importance of sleep and the significance of insufficient sleep, and given that there is strong evidence that people worldwide are not getting enough sleep, you might think that the headlines everywhere would be announcing a "sleep deficiency epidemic" rather than an "obesity epidemic." But clearly, that is not the case. Why might that be? Well, the cynic might suggest that insufficient sleep may be partly attributable to individual choices, but it is far easier to see how industrial and post-industrial cultures and the values of productivity and progress might be called into question should the public begin to examine the sleep issue too closely. Is the cynic right? I don't know. But in any case, whether comfortable or not, we may all benefit greatly by beginning to call into question anything that comes at a higher priority than sufficient sleep.

---

[96] Cappuccio et al., "Meta-analysis of short sleep duration and obesity in children and adults," *Sleep* (May 2008): 619-626.

[97] Nedeltcheva, A.V. et al., "Insufficient Sleep Undermines Dietary Efforts to Reduce Adiposity," *Annals of Internal Medicine* (October 2010): 435-441.

Radiation

It has long been known that large doses of ionizing radiation such as are found in nuclear fallout from weapons or from power plant damage (e.g., Chernobyl) can harm the body in a variety of ways, including cardiovascular disease. In survivors of the atomic attacks on Japan, approximately one third of the deaths are from radiation-related heart disease. Shortly after the Chernobyl accident, a study of exposed humans showed that 18 percent exhibited cardiovascular damage. And those who undergo radiotherapy as a treatment for conditions such as cancer are at significantly greater risk for cardiovascular disease than the rest of the population. What have *not* been studied nearly as well are the effects of *low* doses of ionizing radiation on cardiovascular health.

Ionizing radiation is high-energy, shortwave radiation such as x-rays (found in a lot of medical imaging) and gamma rays (found in nuclear weapons and nuclear power production). Among those who receive the greatest exposure are airline crews, radiographers, medical radiologists, uranium miners, nuclear power workers, and research lab workers. However, over the past decades, the general public has also received significantly greater exposure to ionizing radiation, a matter that we'll look at shortly.

What little research has been done regarding the risk of low-dose ionizing radiation exposure shows that there is indeed a correlation between the dose of radiation and the risk of cardiovascular disease. In a 2009 study,[98] Health Canada reported that the risk of cardiovascular disease among those whose occupations exposed them to regular low doses of ionizing radiation (in the professions previously listed) experience significantly more cases of cardiovascular disease than the rest of the population *and*, significantly, they have higher rates of cardiovascular disease than the survivors of the atomic attack on Japan.

In a meta-analysis published in 2012, the authors concluded that cardiovascular disease risks for those exposed to low levels of ionizing radiation are greater than had previously been thought.[99] And perhaps ironically, a 2011 study[100] demonstrated that low-dose radiation used in cardiology (to examine for heart health) may increase the risk of cardiovascular disease.

Although the amount of research done on the effects of low-dose radiation exposure doesn't allow for any conclusions to be drawn, the picture that is shaping up strongly suggests that there is a connection between ionizing radiation exposure and cardiovascular disease once the radiation dose exceeds some (as of yet undetermined) threshold.

So far, we've seen that those unfortunate enough to live near to a nuclear disaster and those whose occupation exposes them to ionizing radiation are at a higher risk for cardiovascular disease. But what about the general public? Is there any reason to believe that ionizing radiation exposure in the general public could be a contributing factor to heart disease? Unfortunately, there is

---

[98] Zielinski et al., "Low dose ionizing radiation exposure and cardiovascular disease mortality: cohort study based on Canadian national dose registry of radiation workers," *International Journal of Occupational Medicine and Environmental Health* (2009): 27-33.

[99] Little et al., "Systematic review and meta-analysis of circulatory disease from exposure to low-level ionizing radiation and estimates of potential population mortality risks," *Environmental Health Perspective* (November 2012): 1502-1511.

[100] Monceau et al., "Enhanced Sensitivity to Low Dose Irradiation of ApoE−/− Mice Mediated by Early Pro-Inflammatory Profile and Delayed Activation of the TGFβ1 Cascade Involved in Fibrogenesis," *PLoS One* (2013).

presently extremely little research in this matter. However, it is worth considering that general public exposure to ionizing radiation has greatly increased in the past decades.

One of the most common ways in which most people are exposed to ionizing radiation is through medical imaging such as x-rays, CT scans, and PET imaging. A recently published study [101] from the University of California at San Francisco revealed some startling results. The study ran from 1996 to 2010 and each year had between nearly 1 and 2 million people enrolled. Over time they tracked how many medical imaging procedures were being done and how much radiation exposure people were being exposed to. What they found was that the number of procedures has increased, particularly CT scans and PET imaging procedures. Perhaps most importantly, they found that over the fifteen years, the average radiation exposure per person nearly *doubled.*

But medical imaging is not the only way in which exposure has increased over the years. Normally we are all subject to naturally occurring ionizing radiation from various sources, including both the Earth and from cosmic sources. On average, 8 percent of total ionizing radiation exposure is due to cosmic radiation. However, at extreme altitudes, the exposure is much greater, and that is the reason why airline crews receive the greatest dose of ionizing radiation of any profession. Obviously, as already seen, occupational exposure for airline crews is extremely significant. And while I know of no research demonstrating links between passenger hours and risk of cardiovascular diseases, it is reasonable to assume there may be a link.

According to data from the International Civil Aviation Organization, passengers on U.S. flights since 1980 have doubled. Perhaps even more shocking is that worldwide, the number of passengers on flights increased from 1.9 billion in

---

[101] Smith-Bindman et al., "Use of Diagnostic Imaging Studies and Associated Radiation Exposure for Patients Enrolled in Large Integrated Health Care Systems, 1996-2010," *Journal of the American Medical Association* (June 2012): 2400-2409.

2004 to just over 3 billion by 2013. The implication is that many members of the general public are likely now receiving more cosmic radiation than they did just decades ago.

Other sources of ionizing radiation account for significantly less of the average person's exposure, but that doesn't mean that they may not be significant. Consumer products, including tobacco, smoke detectors, some watch parts, natural gas, and fluorescent lights (such as compact fluorescent bulbs) account for 3 percent of total ionizing radiation exposure. And radiation exposure from nuclear power production and from coal-fired power plants account for just 1 percent of total average exposure, though, obviously, some people experience much greater exposure than others. Those living closest to power plants and mining operations are at greatest risk.

Thus far, we've looked only at ionizing radiation because that is the type of radiation that has been proven to pose the greatest risk to health. However, another form of radiation, non-ionizing radiation, now exists in increasing levels. Non-ionizing radiation includes many types of radiation such as visible light, infrared, microwave, and radio. Although all forms of radiation exist naturally, human generated non-ionizing radiation has increased dramatically over the past half century. Electrical power transmission, radio and television broadcasting, cell phones, and wireless internet technologies all are examples of human generated non-ionizing radiation.

Unlike ionizing radiation, there does not exist a consensus among researchers that non-ionizing radiation causes harm to human health when exposure is moderate. Of course, in sufficient amounts, non-ionizing radiation is well-known to cause many ill health effects ranging from burning of skin and superficial tissues, damage to eyes, raising the body temperature, damaging nerve and muscle response, and nausea. And in large amounts, it can be fatally toxic. And for this reason, various governmental and non-governmental organizations set limits on how much exposure is allowed to the general public through military or commercial applications or through consumer products.

However, while still not well proven, there is some evidence that chronic low-dose exposure to non-ionizing radiation can have negative health effects. Perhaps the area in which there exists the most agreement regarding the negative impacts of non-ionizing radiation is in regard to the risks to electrical workers. Several studies have found that the greater the magnetic field exposure among electrical workers, the greater the risk of cardiovascular disease.[102] And one of the largest non-ionizing radiation sources (according to the numbers published by the National Radiological Protection Board) is high-tension power lines. Relative to the usual electromagnetic field found outside, the electrical field on the ground directly underneath a 400 kV power line is more than 10,000 times the strength. Within 25 meters of the power line, the field is 1,000 times stronger than the usual field strength. Near domestic appliances (refrigerators, washing machines, etc.) the field strength is between 10 and 250 times as strong. And within a typical home, the field strength is anywhere from slightly stronger to 10 times as strong.

So depending on where one lives (proximity to power lines, number and types of appliances, quality of wiring and shielding, etc.), the normal exposure to electromagnetic fields can be considerably stronger than would be found in most places in nature. It has been suggested that due to the proximity at which some devices are operated to the body, some electrical devices

---

[102] Savitz et al., "Magnetic field exposure and cardiovascular disease mortality among electric utility workers," *American Journal of Epidemiology* (January 1999): 135-142; Van Wijngaarden et al., "Mortality patterns by occupation in a cohort of electric utility workers," *American Journal of Industrial Medicine* (December 2001): 667-673; It's worth noting that another study conducted by J. Sahl & Associates suggested that the risks in the previous two studies were overstated. However, there is reason to believe that J. Sahl, who began a director position with Southern California Edison immediately following the publication of the study may have had a bias.

expose humans to large amounts of non-ionizing radiation despite the relatively small amount of radiation they produce compared to other devices. Examples include hair dryers and electric razors.

The forms of non-ionizing radiation exposure that have proved the most contentious are cell phones (and cell phone infrastructure) and wireless technologies, including digital utility meters (a.k.a. smart meters). There are a growing number of people who believe that these forms of radiation are harmful. However, to date, there is actually no proof that this is so. Most organizations that monitor the effects of such things, including the WHO, have taken a position of carefully monitoring and investigating the effects. In 2011, the WHO issued a press release classifying electromagnetic fields (EMFs) such as those produced by cell phones as *possibly* carcinogenic based on the fact that one type of cancer (glioma) occurs more frequently in those who use cell phones more often.

As soon as the press release was issued, anti-cell phone and anti-wireless groups and individuals started celebrating that they had proof that the technologies are harmful. But it turns out that the classification that the WHO used for electromagnetic fields (Group 2B) is for *possible* carcinogens, a group that also includes aloe vera and ginkgo biloba extract. But then again, the group also includes lead, potassium bromate, vinyl acetate, heptachlor (a heavily restricted insecticide), chloroform, DDT, and over 200 other substances (most of which are chemical names such as 3,3'-Dichloro-4,4'-diaminodiphenyl ether). Basically, Group 2B is for substances that the WHO just can't classify. They *may* be carcinogenic, but then again, they may not. So the classification of EMFs as possible carcinogens means very little.

Regarding non-ionizing radiation, there is some evidence that high exposure may be linked to cardiovascular disease, cancer, and possibly other conditions. However, there is no consensus. As far as the levels at which most people are exposed on a daily basis, the jury is still out. To date, there is no strong evidence that non-ionizing radiation from household electricity, appliances, cell phones, and wireless technology causes health problems for most people. However, since most of the technology in question is quite new and since the levels of exposure are increasing dramatically and rapidly, it is certainly a subject that we would do well to explore more thoroughly. There are practically no well-designed human trials on the subject.

Finally, in the discussion of radiation, it is worth checking to see if there is any evidence that radiation exposure may be connected to increased fatness. It turns out that this is a matter that is now receiving some attention, and the evidence is starting to demonstrate a link. The effects of ionizing radiation exposure in childhood were linked to increased fatness later in life in a study published in the *Journal of Clinical Oncology* in 2003.[103] In that study, it was found that treating children with radiation for cancer was a significant predictor of increased fatness in adulthood. The study was specifically looking at high-dose treatments, so it is not known what links may exist at lower doses, particularly cumulative low doses.

As far as non-ionizing radiation goes, a study published in 2012 [104] found that prenatal exposure to EMFs was clearly correlated with increased fatness in adulthood. The researchers found that the effect was dose dependent, meaning that more EMF exposure correlated with more fatness.

In conclusion, it would seem that the link between radiation exposure and disease is often overlooked. While ionizing radiation seems to have the strongest connection, the dramatic rise in exposure to both ionizing and nonionizing radiation may be reason to give more careful consideration to the potential implications for health.

---

[103] Oeffinger et al., "Obesity in Adult Survivors of Childhood Acute Lymphoblastic Leukemia: A Report from the Childhood Cancer Survivor Study," *Journal of Clinical Oncology* (2003): 1359-1365.

[104] Li et al., "A Prospective Study of In-utero Exposure to Magnetic Fields and the Risk of Childhood Obesity," *Scientific Reports* (July 2012).

Pharmaceuticals

It is no secret that pharmaceutical drug use has been on the rise over the past many decades. According to NHANES data, not only are more Americans using prescription drugs with each passing year, but more people are using *more* drugs; the number of people reporting using five or more prescription drugs at a time continues to increase.

Statins are the most prescribed drug in the world. These drugs lower plasma cholesterol levels, and they normally do so quite well. In fact, looking at the NHANES data, there is a strong correlation between increases in statin prescriptions and decreases in cholesterol levels over time. Because of the presumed causative role of cholesterol in cardiovascular disease (an association that is falling under increasing scrutiny), statins are prescribed to prevent cardiovascular disease and cardiovascular disease events.

Unfortunately, among the known side effects of statins are muscle pain and damage, liver damage, and...diabetes. How big of an increase in risk do statins create for developing diabetes? According to one study,[105] the risk among those using statins may be 27 percent greater than those who don't use statins.

Furthermore, it has been noted that statin users often gain weight. In a study published in the *Journal of the American Medical*

---

[105] Ridker et al., "Rosuvastatin to prevent vascular events in men and women with elevated C-reactive protein," *New England Journal of Medicine* (2008): 2195–2207.

Association, researchers performed a meta-analysis using NHANES data, hoping to understand why weight gain might be seen in statin users. They compared statin users' dietary habits with those of non-users from 1999 to 2010. What they reported is that initially the statin users are eating more over time—both more calories and more fat. Of course, what isn't clear is *why* they are eating more. In the conventional paradigm, it may be tempting to believe that they are getting fatter *because* they are eating more. But it could be that they are eating more because they are getting fatter or that statins or some other factor causes both eating more and weight gain. Given what we have seen in support of setpoint theory, it seems plausible that statins may raise the setpoint, which may require more food.

Statins beat out antidepressants for first place by a very narrow margin, making antidepressants the second most commonly prescribed drug. Antidepressants are generally classified as first generation (monoamine oxidase inhibitors and tricyclic antidepressant drugs) and second generation (selective serotonin reuptake inhibitors (SSRIs) and others).

First-generation antidepressants are notorious for causing cardiovascular problems. Second-generation drugs were said to produce no increased risk, but now it is known that they *do*, in fact, increase cardiovascular risk.[106]

What about diabetes? All classes of antidepressant drugs have been linked with significant increase in the development of type 2 diabetes. In a study published in the *European Journal of Clinical Pharmacology*, the researchers report that tricyclic drugs increase risk by 76 percent while the slightly more benign second-generation drugs increase risk between 37 and 58 percent. A

---

[106] Pacher, P. and Kecskemeti, V., "Cardiovascular Side Effects of New Antidepressants and Antipsychotics: New Drugs, old Concerns?," *Current Pharmaceutical Design* (2004): 2463-2475.

Finnish study[107] also finds that *long-term* use of antidepressant drugs may more than double the risk of developing diabetes.

Antidepressant drugs are well known among users for their association with weight gain. The Finnish study cited in the previous paragraph also found that antidepressant use was strongly correlated with weight gain. In a large-scale meta-analysis,[108] Italian researchers found that weight gain is strongly associated with many, though not all, antidepressant drugs.

Many other popular drugs also are known to produce metabolic changes that could also potentially increase risk of non-communicable diseases, and many drugs are known to produce weight gain. Many anti-diabetes drugs are associated with cardiovascular risk. In fact, one popular drug, Avandia (rosiglitazone), has been withdrawn from several markets because of a meta-analysis[109] that revealed a significant increase in risk of heart attacks associated with the drug. Many anti-diabetes drugs are linked to weight gain,[110] as are hormonal contraceptives, antibiotics, and other popular drugs.

Not only are those who get prescriptions filled potentially at risk, but increasing numbers of pharmaceuticals in the air, land, and water have the potential to increase risk more widely. The U.S. Environmental Protection Agency (EPA) tracks what it calls pharmaceutical and personal care products as pollutants (PPCPs). According to the EPA, "PPCPs comprise a diverse collection of thousands of chemical substances, including prescription and over-the-counter therapeutic drugs, veterinary

---

[107] Kivimaki et al., "Antidepressant Medication Use, Weight Gain, and Risk of Type 2 Diabetes," *Diabetes Care* (December 2010): 2611-2616.

[108] Serretti, A. and Mandelli, L., "Antidepressants and body weight: a comprehensive review and meta-analysis," *Journal of Clinical Psychiatry* (October 2010): 1259-1272.

[109] Nissen, S.E., Wolski, K., "Effect of rosiglitazone on the risk of myocardial infarction and death from cardiovascular causes," *New England Journal Medicine* (2007): 2457–71.

[110] Hollander, P., "Anti-Diabetes and Anti-Obesity Medications: Effects on Weight in People with Diabetes," *Diabetes Spectrum* (July 2007): 159-165.

drugs, fragrances, lotions, and cosmetics," and PPCPs can enter the environment when "medication residues pass out of the body and into sewer lines, externally-applied drugs and personal care products they use wash down the shower drain, and unused or expired medications are placed in the trash." PPCPs are found in nearly all water, including not only ground water and oceans, but also in drinking water.[111]

The EPA and other organizations such as the WHO are quick to point out that the amounts of PPCPs found in drinking water are relatively low and that it is believed that the risk associated with PPCPs in most drinking water may be low. However, they also admit that the effects are poorly studied and that susceptible populations (children, pregnant women, etc.) may be at risk. And some have even speculated that global increases in weight may be attributable to some PPCPs.[112]

Whether the effects of pharmaceuticals are limited to those taking the drugs intentionally or whether the effects may be more widespread due to environmental contamination, the simple fact is that large numbers of people are affected by drugs known to increase the risk of developing cardiovascular disease and/or diabetes, and many of the drugs are also known to increase weight gain.

---

[111] http://www.epa.gov/ppcp/faq.html

[112] Riley et al., "Obesity in the United States – Dysbiosis from Exposure to Low-Dose Antibiotics?," *Frontiers in Public Health* (2013): 69.

Environmental Chemicals

Another major factor that often goes completely ignored in the public discussions regarding type 2 diabetes and cardiovascular disease, among other conditions, is the role of man-made chemicals. The focus is normally so intent on diet that no one says a peep about the implications of the dramatic rise in exposure to various known endocrine disrupting chemicals in populations worldwide. In this section, we'll take a look.

The first group of chemicals of concern are chemicals used in the creation of plastics. It is likely that plastics may pose many threats to health, most of which have not yet been well studied. However, at present, one class of chemicals called phthalates, which are used in many plastics, have started to come under scrutiny.

Phthalates are found in an alarming number and variety of products including cosmetics, PVC pipes (used for water), food packaging and storage containers, fragrances, toys, coatings of pharmaceuticals, adhesives, electronics, detergents, paints, inks, building materials, medical devices, and clothing. In various studies, between 98 and 100 percent of humans have been found to have some phthalates in their bodies. So to say that phthalates are ubiquitous is a bit of an understatement. And while concerns and some legislation have caused some reduction in the use of some phthalates, the use of other phthalates has increased substantially.

Not all phthalates are created equal, of course. Some are more toxic than others. So it may be unnecessarily alarmist to be worried about all phthalates. But given the sheer volume and ubiquity of the chemicals, and given the growing body of evidence linking phthalates to various disease conditions, it also seems naive to simply write them off as harmless.

Phthalates come up more than just about any other class of chemicals in literature on endocrine disruptors. Endocrine disruptors can potentially exert a wide range of influences, but for our discussion, we'll keep it focused on cardiovascular disease and diabetes. In a 2014 study,[113] the researchers found that concentrations of a phthalate called DEHP in the urine of children may indicate greater risk for cardiovascular disease. And several studies from Sweden[114] show that metabolites of phthalates in the elderly correlate to various types of cardiovascular disease.

In a study published in 2007, researchers found that three different phthalate metabolites, when found in participant samples, correlated strongly with insulin resistance in men, and the same lead researcher conducted another study published in 2012[115] that linked urinary concentrations of phthalate metabolites with diabetes in women. In another study from

---

[113] Trasande et al., "Dietary phthalates and low-grade albuminuria in US children and adolescents," *Clinical Journal of the American Society of Nephrology* (January 2014): 100-109.

[114] Lind and Lind, "Circulating levels of bisphenol A and phthalates are related to carotid atherosclerosis in the elderly," *Atherosclerosis* (September 2011): 207-213; Olsen, Lind, and Lind, "Associations between circulating levels of bisphenol A and phthalate metabolites and coronary risk in the elderly," *Ecotoxicology and Environmental Safety* (June 2012): 179-183.

[115] James-Todd et al., "Urinary phthalate metabolite concentrations and diabetes among women in the National Health and Nutrition Examination Survey (NHANES) 2001-2008," *Environmental Health Perspectives* (September 2012): 1307-1313.

Sweden,[116] researchers reported that phthalate metabolites in the elderly are associated with diabetes. In another study,[117] it was found that multiple phthalate metabolites were found in significantly higher concentrations in the urine of women with diabetes. The same correlation has been found among young people as well.

Of course, correlation does not prove causation. We don't know why those who are insulin resistant or diabetic have higher urinary concentrations of phthalate metabolites. It could be that they have a higher exposure or it could be that they simply excrete more. But whatever the case, there clearly is *some* sort of link.

Another chemical often associated with plastic because of its use in some plastics to harden them is BPA (bisphenol A). BPA has come under a great deal of scrutiny in recent years, causing many manufacturers to reduce or eliminate its use in various products. But still, BPA remains ubiquitous in many of our environments. BPA is found in polycarbonate plastics, the linings of many canned foods, and thermal paper and carbonless copy paper, making receipts, tickets, and labels some of the most common sources of exposure. BPA can be transferred to the skin in significant amounts through touch. Furthermore, a paper published in 2011 [118] reported that paper currency can be a significant source of BPA, likely because of frequent contact with BPA paper (i.e., receipts in wallets next to currency). Studies by the CDC and other organizations have consistently found BPA in more than 90 percent of people tested.

In terms of the effects of BPA, the opinions are mixed. Most European and North American agencies involved in regulation

---

[116] Lind, Zethelius, and Lind, "Circulating levels of phthalate metabolites are associated with prevalent diabetes in the elderly," *Diabetes Care* (July 2012): 1519-1524.

[117] Svensson et al., "Phthalate exposure associated with self-reported diabetes among Mexican women," *Environmental Research* (August 2011): 792-796.

[118] Liao and Kannan, "High levels of bisphenol A in paper currencies from several countries, and implications for dermal exposure," *Environmental Science and Technology* (August 2011).

of chemicals in foods and products claim that BPA causes no harm to humans. However, many studies provide evidence that BPA is linked to diseases, including diabetes and cardiovascular disease. Several of the studies cited in reference to phthalates also found that BPA concentrations in urine were linked with diabetes and cardiovascular disease. The U.S. National Toxicological Program reported in 2008 that there is reason for concern about the potential effects of BPA in susceptible populations, including pregnant women and young children. A paper published in *Thyroid* in 2007 reported that BPA can negatively impact thyroid hormones, which can lead to many different conditions. And in 2008, a publication in the *Journal of the American Medical Association*[119] concluded that BPA urinary concentrations were associated with cardiovascular disease and diabetes.

There are lots of other common chemicals that have also been shown to have similarly undesirable effects. Among them are chlorinated and brominated chemicals. Examples of chlorinated chemicals include many glues, cleaners, spray paints, paint strippers, water repellents, mothballs, and deodorizer products. Furthermore, chlorine such as that found in bleach and in chlorinated water (as found in many municipalities) can react with other chemicals in the environment to produce chloroform. In fact, according to the California Environmental Protection Agency, chlorinated water may be one of the major sources of exposure to chloroform for most people. Chlorinated chemicals are also used as flame retardants in furniture and other products. Chlorinated pesticides have *mostly* been banned in the United States and in many other places (though are reportedly still in frequent use in some places), but the effects of these pesticides are still felt today. In fact, one of the most infamous chlorinated chemicals is the pesticide DDT, which has now been shown to be passed down for generations from mother to child.

---

[119] Lang et al., "Association of urinary bisphenol A concentration with medical disorders and laboratory abnormalities in adults," *Journal of the American Medical Association* (September 2008): 1303-1310.

Examples of brominated chemicals include brominated flame retardants (such as PBDE), brominated pool chemicals, and polybrominated vegetable oils (used in some sodas) and pesticides.

Clearly, chlorinated and brominated chemicals are *extremely* common in our environments. Yet unfortunately, very little research has been done specifically on the effects of these chemicals in relation to cardiovascular disease and diabetes. However, what little has been done suggests there may be a link. A paper published in *Interdisciplinary Toxicology* in 2013[120] links both chlorinated and brominated chemicals to cardiovascular disease. And a study published in *Environmental Research* in 2013 found that there may be a link between PBDE levels in children and future cardiovascular disease. The association between brominated chemicals (particularly fire retardants) and diabetes has also been made.[121]

The list of possible chemical contributors to the increases in disease doesn't stop there, of course. But given the surprising lack of published research into the effects of most of those chemicals on human health, unfortunately, in many cases, we'd only be left to speculate.

What is of particular note is that all of the chemicals thus far mentioned, as well as many others, are now classified as obesogens,[122] which are chemicals or substances known to increase fatness. The fact that many of the chemicals that are found to increase fatness are also shown to increase the risk of cardiovascular disease and diabetes suggests that the chemicals

---

[120] Zeliger, H.I., "Lipophilic chemical exposure as a cause of cardiovascular disease," *Interdisciplinary Toxicology* (June 2013): 55-62.

[121] Lim et al., "Association of Brominated Flame Retardants with Diabetes and Metabolic Syndrome in the U.S. Population, 2003–2004," *Diabetes Care* (September 2008): 1802-1807.

[122] Obesogens include many chemicals, among which are antibiotic drugs, pesticides, wood preservatives, perfluorooctanoic acid found in non-stick pans and microwave popcorn bags, organotins found in vinyl, high fructose corn syrup, phthalates, BPA, some brominated chemicals, and some chlorinated chemicals.

may be an underlying link explaining the rise in both diseases *and* fatness worldwide.

What Now?

My hope with this book is that it opens far more questions than it answers. In fact, I hope that very little was answered, because I certainly don't have the answers. But what is clear as soon as one begins to investigate the "obesity epidemic" is that no one else has the answers either. Yet, sadly, we've been told that the answers are known; fatness causes sickness and fat people are fat because they eat too much and move too little.

As a society, we now have a new form of sanctioned bigotry: fat intolerance. Fat intolerance is not helping anyone, and it clearly is hurting some.

While diet and physical activity likely play *some* role in the whole picture, what that role is isn't entirely clear. Furthermore, it is becoming increasingly evident that the role may be much smaller—or at least much different—than we've been told.

Sure, it seems sensible to drink less soda and walk a little more. But will that *really* prevent disease? And perhaps more importantly, is it really true that most people who have developed cardiovascular disease and diabetes were slurping Big Gulps and shoveling down Twinkies by the handful while immobilized in front of the television 24/7? While those activities (or *in*activities) may contribute to health or the lack thereof, with the evidence that we now have before us, it is disingenuous to suggest that that is the total picture.

There are other factors that may be just as significant if not more significant than diet and physical activity. Among those factors is the simple fact that the biggest risk for disease and death is advanced age and the world population is aging. There may be other factors as well, some of which we've explored in this book—stress, lack of sleep, radiation, pharmaceuticals, and environmental chemicals.

Whatever the case, it seems likely that we would do better to investigate with open minds rather than scapegoating people because of the shape and size of their bodies. The truth may be more complicated than pointing a finger at fat people and trying to shame them. It is entirely possible that some of the most significant factors are those that are occurring at a societal level rather than at an individual level. And in any case, we're all in this together. Isn't it high time we began treating one another and ourselves with kindness and open minds?

Get My Future Books FREE

If you enjoyed this book (Hey, if you made it this far it couldn't have been that bad), you'll probably enjoy many of my other books about health and wellness. And you can get all my new releases in health and wellness for free by signing up for my mailing list at www.joeylotthealth.com. It's simple, it's free, and it's totally honest and legitimate. Nothing scammy or spammy or anything else like that (i.e., I won't be trying to sell you The 7 Dirty Underground Top Secret Weird Tricks for Rock Hard Abs or Young Living Oils). It's just about free books for those who appreciate my work, because I appreciate YOU. Simple as that.

Connect with Me

I welcome your questions, comments, and feedback of any kind. Please feel free to email me at joeylott@gmail.com. I am now receiving so many emails that I cannot always reply to each one, but I do read them all, and I do my best to reply to as many as possible. For the benefit of others, I may choose to publish my response to your email on my blog or in book format. I will maintain your privacy and anonymity should I choose to publish my response.

One Small Favor

My sincere goal in writing is to share something that may be of value to you. And I endeavor to do so while keeping the cost low for readers. The success of my books and my ability to reach other readers who may benefit from my books depends in large part on having lots of thoughtful, honest reviews written about my work. You would do me a great favor if you would please take a moment to generously write a review of this book on Amazon.com. This will only take a few minutes of your time, and you will be helping me a great deal. I sure would appreciate it.

About the Author

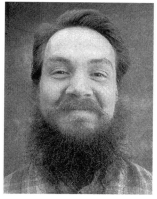

"The secret to happiness is to let go of everything - see through every assumption."

Beginning at a young age Joey Lott experienced intensifying anxiety. For several decades he lived with restrictive eating disorders, obsessions, compulsions, and an inescapable fear. By the time he was 30 years old he was physically sick, emotionally volatile, and mentally obsessed with keeping any and all unwanted thoughts and experiences at bay.

At this time Lott was living on a futon mattress in a tiny cabin in the woods. He was so sick that he could barely move. He was deeply depressed and hopeless. All this despite doing all the "right" things such as years of meditation, yoga, various "perfect" diets, clean air, and pure water.

Just when things were at their most dire, a crack appeared in the conceptual world that had formerly been mistaken for reality. By peering into this crack and underneath all the assumptions that had been unquestioned up to that moment, Lott began a great undoing. The revelation of this undoing is that reality is utterly simple, ever-present, seamless, and indivisible.

Lott's books provide a glimpse into the seamless, simple, and joyous nature of reality, offering a glimpse through the crack in conceptual worlds. Whether writing about the ultimate non-dual nature of reality, eating disorders, stress, disease, or any other subject, he offers the invitation to look at things differently, leaving behind the old, out-grown, painful limitations we have used to bind ourselves in suffering. And then, he welcomes you home to the effortless simplicity of yourself as you are.

Not sure where to begin? Pick up a copy of Lott's most popular book, *You're Trying Too Hard*, which strips away all the concepts that keep us searching for a greater, more spiritual, more peaceful life or self.

Made in the USA
Middletown, DE
03 July 2018